The Killing Field Known as Hospice

Published by Power of the Pen Publishing

His Spirit Fights Back, The premature Death of Steven Lee Hatch,
    July 13, 1948 – August 6, 2015
Involuntary Euthanasia of a Disabled Man is a Vile Form of Homicide
Please Don't Let Me Die! From Stroke to Death in 49 days
Pure, White and Deadly, How Sugar is Killing Us and What We Can Do
    to Stop It. By Dr. John Yudkin.
Shortcut to Heaven, Why Death With Dignity Legislation is Needed Now
Strokes Can Be Deadly If You Have the Wrong Doctors
Stroke Victims Have Rights, All About Strokes and Recovery
The Dilemmas of Euthanasia Edited by John A. Behnke and Sissela Bok
The Vigilante of Nemaha, Iowa One Woman's Crusade to Protect
    a Small Town
There Must Be an Easier Way to Die
Trust No One! The Doctors Responsible for the Death of Steven Lee Hatch
    August 6, 2015
Vermont Folk Medicine by Dr. D.C. Jarvis, Second Edition, enlarged

The Killing Field Known as Hospice

By Marlys J. Waters

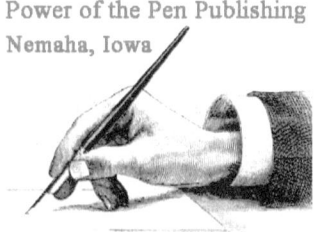

Power of the Pen Publishing
Nemaha, Iowa

Copyright 2018 by Marlys J. Waters

ISBN-13: 978-1985068711

ISBN-10: 1985068710

Published by:
Power of the Pen Publishing
PO Box 5
Nemaha, IA 50567

Printed in the United States of America

Dedication

I dedicate this fact-finding document to Steven L Hatch, the man that made my life complete. I had known Steve since we were kids but became the best of friends after retirement age when we became a couple.

After Steve's death 49 days following a stroke suffered June 21, 2015, I became co-administrator of his estate giving me access to his medical records. Two years later I wrote this story of why he died. You will not believe what you read. You may even have doubts that the medical profession is actively killing people who they believe have no worth.

Before you close this book on Steve's Life and Death, you might want to also read "The Dilemmas of Euthanasia" edited by John A. Behnke and Sissela Bok which I have republished in larger print on studies completed in 1975 on involuntary euthanasia. Steve's death is not an isolated case, people are being euthanized all over and most people don't realize why their loved one died.

Another book written by Ron Panzer in 2011 titled "Stealth Euthanasia" presents other horror stories from people who share the loss of their loved ones while in hospice. Ron worked as a nurse and in hospice. He exposes how low the medical profession has digressed to shuffle the elderly and weak people into hospice where they are killed for profit.

No legal entity at local, state, or federal level will investigate reports of "involuntary euthanasia", aka murder of defenseless people while in hospice. The deaths are escalating. Getting people out of Medicare pays quite well. Large hospice corporations are well reimbursed for their work.

As of 02/03/2018 I have not heard back from any agency willing to work on my claim that a murder was committed. Pay attention because you are living in this world and you might be their next victim!

Table of Contents

Introduction	1
Summary of Care at Loring Hospital on 06/21/15	3
Summary of Aspiration Pneumonia at Mercy Medical Center	4
Summary of Care at Mercy Medical Center	15
Blackhawk Life Care Center and Gentiva Hospice - Second Hospice Attempt	17
Iowa State Hospice Rules 2015	21
Blackhawk Hawk Life Care – Second Aspiration Incident	23
Loring Hospital Critical Care 07/16/15 – 07/20/15	25
About Steve's Fractured Skull at age 6 on May 2, 1955	29
Blackhawk Life Care Center – Narcotics/Opioids 07/07/15 – 07/16/15	31
Steve Hatch Was Successfully Treated at Loring Hospital For Aspiration Pneumonia	39
Loring Hospital - Excessive Meds Over Extra Four Days	41
Lethal Medications Given During Steve's Final 13 Days	52
Doctors Who Worked Against Steve's Best Interest	57
Leading to His Death	57
The Admittance into Gentiva Hospice 07/24/15	71
Was a Profitable move for them	71
About the Author	73

Introduction

My twelve-year companion, Steven Lee Hatch, age 67, was involuntarily euthanized in hospice with excessive and lethal medications 49 days after suffering a stroke. The stroke had left him paralyzed on one side and unable to swallow or to speak other than to answer "yes" and "no". Steve's death took place at Blackhawk Life Care Center in Lake View, Sac County, Iowa on August 6, 2015, just 13 days after he had been forced into Hospice on July 24, 2015 without his consent or knowledge at Loring Hospital in Sac City. He did not have a terminal illness and he had refused admittance into hospice verbally in front of 4 witnesses on 7/8/2015.

According to Iowa State law, a person who is conscious can not be legally admitted into hospice against their will and without having a terminal illness. The majority of people who suffer strokes survive. Strokes take weeks to months before improvement with proper therapy can be seen. Steve was forced into hospice just one month after suffering the stroke.

Steve Hatch needed a chance at stroke therapy and rehabilitation. If recovery of his lost abilities was not possible after a period of time and his health declined, then he could have requested admittance into hospice at a later date. There was no rush. The stroke had stabilized with no further change in the head scans/x-rays. He had Medicare, supplemental insurance, and cash assets for the best stroke rehabilitation available.

Steve had other long-term disorders that he had been living with for over 12 years which he was able to control with one or two pills a day for diabetes, aortic stenosis (reduction of blood flow from the heart), COPD, and high blood pressure.

Steve's final job had been at a turkey processing plant for thirteen years ending in 2003 where the diesel fumes from the trucks had affected his lungs causing him to be placed on Social Security disability due to irreversible lung damage at age 55. The COPD caused a need to avoid dust, mold, smoke, and any activity that required strenuous walking. He also slept with a nasal cannula delivering 2 LPM oxygen but didn't need external oxygen during the day time unless he was suffering from a temporary illness like a common cold.

Steve was a very active, outdoor farm man. While he cash-rented most of his farm ground, he kept the hay ground for his own use, cut and baled hay using antique tractors and equipment that he maintained. He also mowed lawns on over 10 acres. He planted a huge garden every year, canned and froze the majority of the produce, and raised a few pigs to have butchered for pork. He also cut down hollow, dying trees on two farmsteads. He could do most stationary tasks as long as he could take frequent rest breaks and avoid fumes, smoke, dust, and mold.

The medical professionals were reluctant to give Steve Hatch the rehabilitation he needed through therapy for his paralyzed right arm and leg, and for speech/swallowing therapy to regain his voice and swallowing reflux which had been temporarily disrupted by the stroke.

Instead, Steve was subjected to sedation by narcotics which depressed his heart and lung function. He was left with an NG (naso-gastric) tube for 8 days through his nose, down his throat into his stomach for nutrients and medications which was susceptible to fluids backing up into his lungs.

Leaving that tube in his throat for eight days also interfered with any chance for receiving exercises/therapy to regain his ability to swallow and speak.

My name is Marlys J. Waters, author of this publication. I was Steve's companion for 12 years. I had known Steve, his brothers, his parents and grandparents since the 1950s after having grown up in the same rural Iowa countryside.

I accompanied Steve to all of his doctor appointments during the 12 years we were together (2003 – 2015). I helped him register with the best supplemental medical insurance available. I also have a lot of experience taking care of sick people. I could have taken care of him at home but wasn't given the chance. We had to wait for a judge to grant me legal Guardian/Conservator status with the approval of Steve's brother. A court date was set for August 10, 2015, four days AFTER he was involuntarily euthanized with Lortab and Morphine.

This photo was taken at Loring Outpatient in 2013 while waiting for blood transfusions needed for GI bleeding caused by Zafirlukast (ACCOLATE), a medication prescribed for breathing which caused almost two years of GI-bleeding and multiple hospitalizations. Steve and I had to solve that mystery to save his life.

Summary of Care at Loring Hospital on 06/21/15

The evening of 06/20/415 we ate supper together but Steve wasn't very hungry. He had spent 5 hours mowing so was hot, tired, and sunburned. I also was worn out after I had picked up sticks ahead of the riding lawnmower. I could barely stay ahead of him as he hadn't given me much advance notice that he was planning to mow that day.

The next morning I found him on the carpeted floor of his bedroom. Steve was lying on his right (paralyzed) side making eye contact but not speaking. He was reaching over his head with his left arm trying to turn the floor fan off. I was unable to get him up so realized something was wrong and called for an ambulance.

The First Responders arrived at the house within minutes followed by the ambulance within 20 minutes. They had him at Loring Hospital at Sac City, Iowa emergency room by 0840. He reportedly had some intermittent responses to questions according to EMA (Emergency Medical Ambulance personnel) with occasional nods to questions and squeezing of others hand using his left hand only. He was not able to speak.

Steve Hatch was examined in the ER at Loring by Dr. Bender.

- 06/21/15 11:29 History of Present Illness, report sent to Mercy Medical Center with Ambulance: The patient presents with altered mental status, confusion. was found on the floor of his bedroom by his girlfriend (Marlys Waters) at 0730 this morning with right side weakness and unable to speak. She called EMS and he was taken to Loring Hospital in Sac City.
- 06/21/15 He has some wheezes and rales, he has COPD, and he had been given an albuteral Nebulizer treatment earlier this morning about 0900. The ER doctor - Dr. Bender in Sac City reports that on R.A. on admission the Patient has 02 stats of 89-92% but when put on 2 L/NC he maintained saturation in mid 90's. There is no history of past stroke but he did suffer a brain injury at age 6. His significant other of 12 years drove to Sac City but will not be going to Mercy Hospital in Sioux City today. Same ambulance crew took him to Mercy Medical Center in Sioux City and reported that he seemed weaker and less responsive than he did earlier today.

[I also noticed Steve was no longer making eye contact while still at Loring. MJW]

4   The Killing Field Known as Hospice

Summary of Aspiration Pneumonia at Mercy Medical Center

The first aspiration incident occurred at Mercy Medical Center in Sioux City on 06/23/15 just two days after the stroke. It was caused by caregiver negligence in giving an unsafe volume of liquid nutrients through an NG (nasogastric) tube as he lay flat on his back in bed. The stomach liquid backed up into his lungs over a period of 24 hours indicated by increasing difficulty breathing as noted by the admitting doctor and nurses in the stroke ward who were monitoring him.

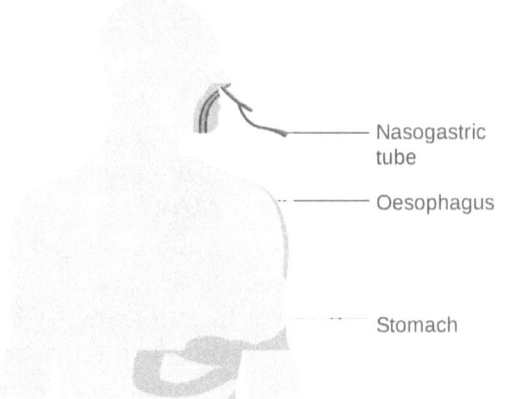

Steve went unresponsive (unconscious) due to lack of oxygen to the brain called hypoxia (he drowned due to caregiver error). A doctor was paged and Steve was transferred to the ICU and revived by intubation requiring sedation to suck the fluids out of his lungs.

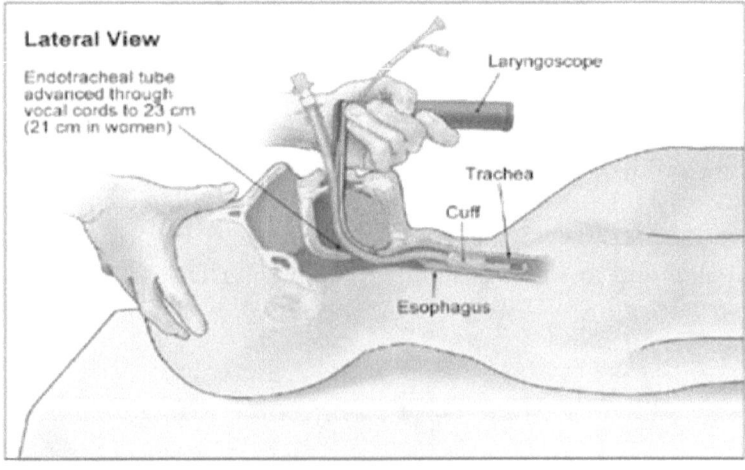

A week later they placed a safer PEG-tube for feedings and medications. The **P**ercutaneous **E**ndoscopic **G**astrostomy tube is a flexible feeding tube placed through the abdominal wall and into the stomach. The procedure requires minimal sedatives and a couple of days recovery as the sutures heal.

The PEG-tube allows nutrition, fluids and/or medications to be put directly into the stomach, bypassing the mouth and esophagus of persons who are temporarily unable to swallow. It can easily be monitored using a large syringe to measure the amount of stomach residue before subsequent feeding bags are hooked up for gravity feedings.

The PEG-tube does not interfere with the stomach sphincter muscle which keeps stomach contents from backing up into the esophagus unlike the NG tube which holds the sphincter muscle open. However the sphincter valve opens voluntarily in the case of vomiting.

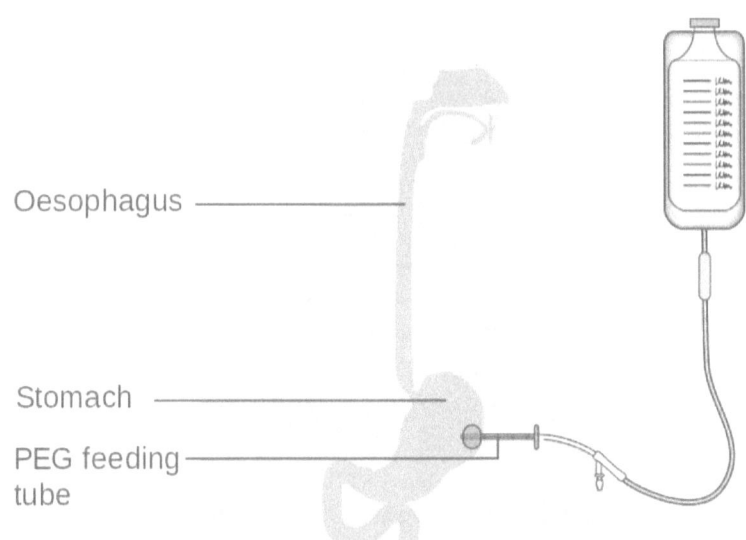

So even with a PEG-tube, the patient who is unable to swallow or is partially paralyzed and unable to roll over to get their head over a bucket can still aspirate stomach fluids into the lungs. Many medications irritate the stomach and cause vomiting. Steve's second and third aspiration incidents at a different facility will be caused by sedatives/opioids which induced vomiting causing his lungs to fill with stomach contents over separate periods of 4-5 days each time.

There is a direct cause and effect shown in the medical records indicating where Steve had increasing trouble breathing following administration of sedatives/opioids/narcotics. Can you imagine the terror experienced by a person paralyzed on one side, unable to speak as his lungs are slowly filling with liquid? All while trying to stay awake from the sedatives?

Mercy Medical Center's solution was to cover his nose and mouth with an oxy-mask which was delivering oxygen of higher concentration than normal room air. Then they tied his left (non-paralyzed) arm to the bed rail so he couldn't pull the face mask off. They placed an oxygen monitor on his finger to record the continuous oxygen level in the blood.

What would be your reaction if you were flat on your back in a bed, had no way to get up, roll over, or call for help and were having great difficulty breathing? You know the face mask is not working at keeping your blood oxygen at a safe level but you don't know why so you try to pull it off. *[Steve was having trouble breathing so he was trying to get the plastic face mask (oxymask) off thinking that is what is interfering with his breathing. MJW]*

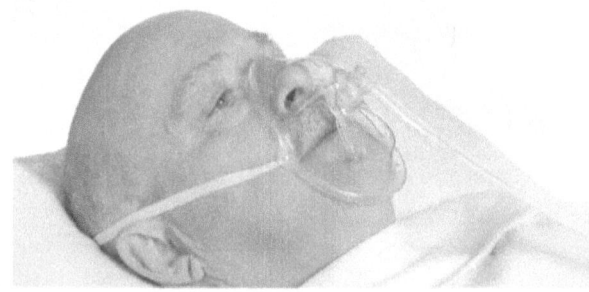

Example of an oxymask covering nose, mouth, and chin hooked to concentrated oxygen source. Open concept delivers concentrated oxygen to both nose and mouth (for mouth breathers). Side openings allow CO_2 to escape when exhaling or for expelling vomit.

The nurses who were monitoring his blood oxygen through the oxygen monitor knew his blood-oxygen count was going down, heart rate was increasing at an alarming rate trying to circulate the blood faster to get the dwindling oxygen supply to all parts of the body and specifically to the brain. So what did the nurses do?

The nurses did nothing for 24 hours other than to tie Steve's left arm to the bed frame and to warn him that he was NOT supposed to pull the face mask off. They didn't even have the foresight to elevate the head of the bed to allow gravity to slow down the horizontal movement of fluids from his stomach into his lungs.

Timeline by date/hour

➢ 06/22/15 0844 Dr. Shaheer Siddiqui examined Steve in ICU. "Yesterday he was absolutely unresponsive in ER (emergency room) but today he is opening eyes on verbal commands and is able to answer my questions via yes or no and he is understanding what I am saying. The patient is lying in bed on <u>flat bed rest</u>." "The Patient is having trouble ventilating as indicated by abdominal breathing."

["Flat Bed Rest" is a poor position for an overweight, paraplegic man with COPD and unable to speak/swallow with a nasogastric tube through his nose down his throat into his stomach. The sphincter muscle at the top of the stomach would not be able to close completely to keep stomach fluids from backing up into his esophagus where they could be inhaled into his lungs – which is what happened. MJW].

Dr. Siddiqui had been the first person to notice Steve was having trouble breathing. Follow the "trail of fools" who continue to record and do nothing about his increasing difficulty breathing.

- 06/22/15 13:00 Patient transferred to stroke ward.
- 06/22/15 17:30 Patient arrived in stroke ward with left wrist restraint. Pt is impulsive and tries to reach at his face.
- 06/23/15 02:49 Feedings restarted at a very low rate.
- 06/23/15 05:01 Feedings turned up.
- 06/23/15 06:42 Seems dyspnec. *[Having trouble breathing. MJW]*
- 06/23/15 12:16 Dr. Elizabeth Hartman: Patient was transferred out of the ICU to the Stroke Unit. Mental status: Opens eyes to voice, tracks examiner, attempts to state his name and age but is dysarthric. Echocardiogram did not reveal any significant changes compared to 01/2013. *[Dysarthria often is characterized by slurred or slow speech that can be difficult to understand. Common causes of dysarthria include nervous system (neurological) disorders such as stroke and conditions that cause facial paralysis of tongue or throat muscle weakness. MJW]*
- 06/23/15 19:35:Feeding stopped due to high residual of 100cc. Refed. *[Residual indicates he did not finish digesting the previous feeding. Within 90 minutes after feedings, at least 50% of the contents of your stomach should already have emptied into the small intestine. Food that stays in the stomach too long can ferment, which can lead to the growth of bacteria and/or cause vomiting – very dangerous for a paralyzed man laying flat on his back and who is unable to swallow. MJW]*
- 06/23/15 21:30: Feeding was restarted. *[Feeding was restarted 2 hours later with no relief or examination for his increasing labored breathing. MJW]*
- 06/23/15 22:40 Patient very agitated at this time. *[Agitated because he can't breathe as his lungs continue to fill up with fluid. MJW]*

- 06/24/15 00:35 Patient <u>heart rate 106 to 176 at times</u>, Patient very restless and constantly moving left (non-paralyzed) side. *[His heart rate is racing due to lack of oxygen. Ignoring his breathing crisis is cruel and inhumane treatment of a paralyzed man who can't speak. MJW]*
- 06/24/15 04:29: Patient becoming increasingly restless, sounding wheezy, and lungs crackles and coarse. Dr. Paged. *[Doctor finally paged due to patient breathing difficulty. Excess fluid in lungs can cause bibasilar (2-sided) crackles detectable with a stethoscope. MJW]*
- 06/24/15 04:50: Patient continues to struggle to breathe, Dr. paged and request for patient to transfer to ICU: Patient arrives at ICU room 5132, restless and dyspnec, using accessory muscles. Respiratory Therapist placed BiPAP, Arterial blood gas drawn, chest x-ray completed. Patient breathing easier on BiPAP, feedings and IV stopped. Nasogastric Tube placed to low intermittent <u>suction</u> of stomach contents. *[More than 24 hours elapsed since Steve became dyspnec as noted by Dr. Shaheer Siddiqui who left no cautions to nursing staff to monitor his breathing and heart rate. Feedings were restarted causing patient undue suffering as his labored breathing and restlessness were recorded but ignored while his lungs continued to fill with stomach contents (vomit) and he went unresponsive from lack of oxygen to the brain. This is incompetent doctoring and nursing to allow a paralyzed patient to <u>drown</u> in the 4-bed stroke ward with 24-hour onsite nursing staff in attendance. MJW]*
- 06/24/15 14:27 Dr. Thomas Murphy was called when Steve had a respiratory event in the stroke ward, secondary to aspiration of tube feedings. He was wet and gurgling and had significant rhonchi, rales and wheezes. He is in acute respiratory failure. Social work will discuss care with brother.
- 06/24/15 14:27 Dr. Thomas Murphy examined Steve and reported: Pt. regained consciousness after being **intubated** in the ICU (intensive care unit) at Mercy Hospital.
- 06/24/15 19:36: Dr. Murphy in unit, talks with patient's brother about diagnosis, plan of care. Questions asked and answered. *[As Steve's Significant Other of 12 years and having been involved in Steve's health care during those years, I was completely excluded from all discussions on his prognosis and future plans. This omission of forcing Steve to be sent through the medical journey alone and not*

being able to make his own decisions while temporarily disabled by a stroke goes against all compassion for what the patient wanted.
➢ 06/25/15 09:06 Dr. Shaheer Siddiqui. Patient examined in ICU. Little more responsive, able to follow commands and now speak a few words. He is extremely anxious. Physical Therapy, Occupational therapy, and Speech Therapy will be working with patient. *[Respiration rate of 47 is quite fast. MJW]*
➢ 06/25/15 13:38 Dr. Thomas Murphy. May need feeding tube placed. If he aspirates again, I would recommend that he either gets a tube feeding or may need a trach. It may be beneficial to make him a do not resuscitate if he continues to aspirate. *[Steve aspirated due to the NG tube through his nose allowing his lungs to fill up with fluid over 24 hours of neglect. It was staff error, don't kill the man just because you made a mistake. Dr. Murphy thinks Steve should not be resuscitated if it happens again. MJW]*
➢ 06/26/15 11:05 Dr. Jon A. Peacock. Patient aspirated Tuesday night 06/24/15. Prognosis is very guarded. A brother is hopefully coming to discuss code status and further options for treatment.
➢ 06/26/15 12:17 Dr. James L. Case, Neurology service. He is on Precedex, lightly sedated. *[Precedex is for awake fiberoptic intubation in adult patients. MJW]* I have consulted Dr. Elizabeth McInerney of palliative care who will speak with patient's brother.
➢ 06/26/15 13:50 Dr. Thomas Murphy. We have taken him off the BiPAP. He has CO2 retention *[Carbon dioxide retention is a symptom of hypoxia or lack of oxygen to the brain. MJW]*. He is on Precedex for rate control and on insulin drip. Not able to lay still enough for CT of his head. Would hold off on nutrition unless he tolerates being off the BiPAP mask. **We are having some issues waking him up.** Ordered Fentanyl *[Fentany is roughly 100 times more potent than morphine and 50 times more potent than heroin. In fact, it is the most potent opioid pain reliever available for use in medical treatment. Also ordered was Haldol, an antipsychotic medicine. If you have high blood sugar (diabetes), you will need to watch your blood sugar closely. Sudden death and heartbeats that are not normal have happened with Haldol. If you are 65 or older, use this medicine with care. You could have more side effects. MJW]*
➢ 06/26/15 14:04 Dr. Shaheer Siddiqui. Patient seen in ICU, is on Precedex drip because he was extremely agitated. He is on BiPAP support. Currently lethargic and unresponsive. Lungs clear via stethoscope.

➤ 06/26/15 16:54 Dr .Elizabeth McInerney, Dr. James Case (consulting physician). Transferred to ICU with aspiration pneumonia on 06/24/15. Discussion with patient's brother. We decided he will be "do not resuscitate" status but all other medical measures are to be undertaken. We would continue to encourage family to consider comfort care at this time due to <u>grim prognosis</u> for ever being independent again, necessity for multiple medical interventions. *[If Steve had adequate medical care he wouldn't need multiple medical interventions. MJW]*

➤ 06/27/15 08:51 Dr. Shaheer Siddiqui. Patient still on the BiPAP with Precedex drip so is unresponsive. Patient is sedated, is probably having ileus (vomiting) as lot of secretions out of NG tube which is on suction. Hope to start feeding with Glucerna through NG tube. Patient's prognosis is guarded, high risk of decompensation (deterioration). If NG tube feedings not tolerable, we may place a central line for TPN (Total Parenteral Nutrition feeding that bypasses the gastrointestinal tract where fluids are given into a vein needed nutrients.)

➤ 06/27/15 10:08 Dr. Jon A. Peacock. Patient aspirated Tuesday night (06/24/15 14:27) and currently is NPO (nothing by mouth) and **intubated** in ICU. Diltizaem drip had been discontinued <u>**due to slow heart rates yesterday**</u>. Prognosis is guarded. He is now DNR status and family is contemplating palliative care.

➤ 06/27/15 12:09 Dr. Thomas Murphy, CT Head w/o Contrast compared to prior study of 06/23/15. Unchanged, mass effect appears slightly improved. Changes in widening of the posterior horn of the left lateral ventricle with surrounding edema has not changed.

➤ 06/27/15 12:56 Dr. Thomas Murphy. Overnight patient had to be put back on BiPAP. Was able to get a CT scan while sedated on Precedex drip. No change in intracranial hemorrhage. We continue to treat for aspiration event from tube feedings. We have been able to prevent him from being intubated. *[One doctor said he HAD been intubated which might be confusion over the BiPAP and NG tube hookups. MJW]* He is now DNAR (Do Not Attempt Resuscitation in case of cardio/pulmonary arrest). *[The DNR/DNAR only applies if both his heart and lungs have stopped. MJW]* We will start tube feeds at 10 cc an hour and need to keep head of bed at 30-45 degrees. We may need to have a G-tube placed. *[YES, you need to get the PEG-tube in before he aspirates again. MJW]* **I certainly would not bring him back down to the Intensive Care Unit.** *[Stated Dr. Thomas*

Murphy twice. Doctor Murphy is on precarious legal grounds when he states that Steve Hatch should not be brought back to the Intensive Care Unit again. Follows are the Medicare Federal rules. MJW]

The Emergency Medical Treatment and Active Labor Act (EMTALA) is an act of the United States Congress, passed in 1986 as part of the Consolidated Omnibus Budget Reconciliation Act (COBRA). It requires hospital Emergency Departments that accept payments from Medicare to provide an appropriate medical screening examination (MSE) to individuals seeking treatment for a medical condition, regardless of citizenship, legal status, or ability to pay. There are no reimbursement provisions. **Participating hospitals may not transfer or discharge patients needing emergency treatment except with the informed consent or stabilization of the patient or when their condition requires transfer to a hospital better equipped to administer the treatment.**

- 06/28/15 14:56 Dr. Shaheer Siddiqui. Patient still in ICU, is off the BiPAP and on nasal cannula *[Easier to tolerate nasal cannula without the forced air pressure of the BiPAP. MJW]* Dr. Mei He returns to service tomorrow.
- 06/28/15 16:17 Dr. Thomas Murphy. Respiratory failure secondary to regurgitation/aspiration of tube feedings. Tolerating feedings with head of bed up. Need speech therapy evaluation. May need PEG tube. No significant change in CT scan *[Stoke damage unchanged. MJW]* Going to decrease steroids and bump up insulin. *[Steroids for breathing work against diabetes control. See Loring Hospital records 07/20/15 - 07/24/15 to see what Doctor Leszak Marczewski prescribed for Steve over four days rather than to release him back to the nursing home. MJW]* Haldol as needed. He had been off BiPAP all day, using nasal cannula at 1Lpm.
- 06/29/15 10:02 Dr. Thomas Murphy. Patient is more awake today. Due for PEG tube for feeding today because of swallowing difficulties. Currently has an NG tube. Will be transferred out of ICU and to the medical floor or to Stroke unit on the 8th floor. Tube feed on hold for possible PEG. Patient pulmonary improved significantly. Been off BiPAP since yesterday morning. No respiratory distress, follows commands. He did not have diagnosed sleep apnea but may have that at nighttime. Make sure of continuous oximeter. Was on room air at one point yesterday. Able to stick his tongue out straight. Lungs are clear. 1+ edema in lower extremities and has SCDs in place (Sequential Compression Device shaped like sleeves that wrap around

the legs and inflate one at a time to prevent blood clots.) Plan is for PEG per Dr. Mei He from Neurology.
- 06/29/15 10:07 Dr. Mei He: Patient tolerated extubation, now on face mask for oxygen. Patient following commands, currently improving. Brother agrees with feeding tube. Patient is DNR/DNI. There will be no re-intubation. *[I disagree, the signed DNR document does not have a check mark by "no intubation". MJW]* Going to continue supportive treatment.
- 06/29/15 11:47 Dr. Michael V. Persaud, DO. We have been asked to place a gastrostomy tube because he is unable to swallow without aspirating. Will stop tube feedings at midnight and place PEG tube in a.m.
- 06/29/15 16:59 Dr. Prashanth Garshakurthi. Patient able to follow commands, nods his head. Scheduled for PEG tube placement in a.m. Patient is non-verbal. Is being transferred to Neuro floor.
- 06/30/15 20:35 Dr. Prashanth Garshakurthi: Patient not verbal today given influence of sedation. He received PEG tube placement. Nursing staff reports he was following commands and awake all day. PEG tube site neat, secured with abdominal binder. Left arm restrained with mitten for safety of PEG tube. Cat scan shows intracranial hemorrhage, surrounded by edema which is unchanged. Discharge plan, patient <u>will benefit from rehab</u>, so we will request inpatient rehabilitation consult tomorrow.
- 07/01/15 11:44 Dr. Mei He: Post PEG tube placement, tolerated procedure. Patient sitting up in bed per help of physical Therapy. Was able to look around. Difficulty talking. Right upper extremity has no movement, but rest of the 3 extremities he moves per command. Has some difficulty with tolerating the feedings. The social worker is working on getting patient placement.
- 07/01/15 19:48 Dr. Prashanth Garshakurthi. Evaluated patient in Stroke Unit. He is comfortable and voices response (though slurred) that he is comfortable. Tolerance to Physical Therapy has been suboptimal (below par). NG tube has been removed. Left arm restrained with mitten for safety of PEG tube. Start using the PEG tube for feedings, Glucerna at 50 cc an hour
- 07/02/15 15:05 Dr. Prashanth Garshakurthi. Patient is disoriented, kinda indicates by nodding his head, not in any distress, able to follow simple commands with unaffected left side. Tolerating PEG tube feeds well, almost at goal rate. Peg tube side secured with abdominal binder.

By Marlys J. Waters

Dense hemiplegia (paralysis) on right side. Long holiday weekend, case manager Tammy predicts placement delayed for next 3 days.
- 07/03/15 19:37 Dr. Prashanth Garshakurthi: Evaluated patient in stroke unit. Patient indicates feeling better, no complaints. Tolerating tube feeds very well, remains afebrile (temperature normal), hemodynamically stable (no difficulty with blood circulation), no distress. Renal function (kidneys) improved.
- 07/04/15 11:51 Dr. Prashanth Garshakurthi. Evaluated patient in Stroke Unit. Denies any discomfort. Speech is slurred. No distress. Bilateral air entry improving, getting bronchodilator treatments. Normal vesicular breath sounds. Will change feeds to bolus rate per nutritionist. Anticipating placement to nursing home/skilled care facility early next week.
- 07/05/15 15:22. Dr. Prashanth Garshakurthi. Evaluated patient in Stroke Unit. Patient denys any complaints. Tried to mouth his response, has slurred speech, seems comfortable, tolerating feeds well. Trace pedal edema (accumulation of fluid in the feet and lower legs). Anticipating discharge to skilled care facility in 1-2 days.
- 07/06/15 13:53 Dr. Elizabeth A. McInerney. Patient has improved, mostly awake and alert, comfortable. Palliative care is going to sign off case. DNR was signed but family decided to go with tube feeding and nursing home option. Prognosis extremely guarded, has had several strokes *[Not true. MJW]*, extremely avoidant of all aggressive medical intervention *[Not true. MJW]* and consistently refusing treatment for aortic stenosis over several years.

[NOTE BY MARLYS: DR. Elizabeth A. McInerney twists facts and changes figures just to sign up people into palliative care aka hospice. Steve has NOT had <u>several</u> strokes, He has NOT avoided aggressive medical intervention, and he had NOT refused treatment for his aortic stenosis over several years, just during 2 years when he had undiagnosed GI bleeding. Steve Hatch was hospitalized multiple times between 2013-2014 for unexplained GI bleeding which the specialists and doctors at Mercy Medical Center and at Loring Hospital were unable to solve the source of the bleeding.

Steve's gastro/intestinal bleeding was caused by Zafirlukast (ACCOLATE) prescribed by Dr. Robert Stewart, pulmonary specialist from Mercy Medical Center. Steve and I figured out which medication was causing the problem from a <u>do-not-use</u> book published by the FDA warning of "ulcerative colitis". Per our suggestion Dr. Pek replaced ACCOLATE with something safer and the bleeding stopped within a couple of weeks. It *was during those two years that Steve was too weak for heart surgery and other aggressive medical interventions that were being proposed by the specialists who didn't care that he was having a life-threatening problem caused by one of **their** medications.*

Don't blame Steve for hesitating to put his life in control of doctors who are unable to read medical journals that had been warning against Zafirlukast use since the 1990s. Maybe it was the Zafirlukast (ACCOLATE) prescribed by Dr. Robert Stewart which caused his Afib and aortic stenosis in the first place leading to the stroke. MJW]

More comments regarding statements made about Steve by Dr. Elizabeth A. McInerney on her first encounter with Steve are continued below. *[By Marlys Waters: Dr. Elizabeth A. McInerney lied about meeting with the Significant Other. She didn't even know my name and didn't know Steve had a Significant Other until I showed up to visit Steve and found Don and Mary Ellen Hatch being counseled by her in Mercy Medical Center ICU beside Steve's bed where he lay unconscious.*

Dr. Elizabeth A. McInerney recommended palliative care but didn't mention to the brother that in palliative care there would be NO stroke recovery/rehabilitation or curative care for prior medical issues. All she wanted was to get him out of acute care at Mercy Medical Center. That is probably what she is being paid to do. And that is why people are dying even if they don't have a terminal illness. A recent stroke is not a terminal illness and most people recover.

Some people who are recovering from drowning like Steve can drift in and out of consciousness. Dr. McInerney had no right to be telling the brother right in front of Steve that there was no chance for recovery and it would be best if Steve be put into palliative/comfort care (hospice) and to sign a Do Not Resuscitate order in case of Cardio/pulmonary arrest. Steve may very well have been listening to the conversation. There were several doctors who recognized that even through Steve appeared to be sleeping or sedated, that when they spoke directly to him, he would answer or nod his head at times even when he didn't open his eyes. MJW.]

- ➢ 07/06/15 15:17 Dr. Ashar Luqman, Dr. Shaheer Siddiqui; Patient was supposed to go to skilled nursing facility in Lake View but due to transportation (ambulance) issues, he will be staying overnight at Mercy Medical Center. Medication reconciliation was discharged around 10:00 am. He is ready to be discharged. Patient was awake and alert, no acute distress. Pupils equal and reactive to light. Patient is stable to be transferred tomorrow morning.

By Marlys J. Waters

Summary of Care at Mercy Medical Center

In the first four days at Mercy Medical Center in Sioux City, Iowa following the stroke, the doctors attempted to convince the estranged brother that Steve Hatch had no chance of ever recovering from the stroke. They recommended palliative or comfort care (sedatives, aka hospice) for pain, restlessness, and depression until death. They based their assumption on his being unable to speak which they believed meant no cognitive powers, (brain-dead, comatose, stroke had caused too much damage) and the fact that he had gone unconscious from hypoxia (lungs filled with fluid causing lack of oxygen to the brain from incompetent feedings through a nasogastric tube.)

Staff at Mercy Medical Center did not admit their technical error in allowing a temporarily paralyzed patient to aspirate due to their neglect. So what do they do at Mercy Medical Center next? Read on, it just gets more bizarre by the minute. Pay attention because we are looking at a felony charge of "involuntary euthanasia".

After a stroke, throat muscles often suffer temporary paralysis just like the arms and legs do. Many stroke survivors are first unable to speak or to swallow. Only the family knows if their family member that has been temporarily silenced is still in there. Families base their non-medical analysis on watching eye movement, watching reactions when a familiar face walks in the room and is offered a handshake from the paralyzed patient. They also can recognize a smile even if it is lopsided from the one-sided paralysis after they have told the patient a joke or a funny story.

The early morning hours of 06/24/15 Steve was put into ICU, intubated to suction the fluid out of his lungs, sedated so he wouldn't fight the tubes which also slowed down his breathing,

Just two days later on 06/26/15 Steve was put into DNR status (Do not resuscitate if in cardio/pulmonary arrest). That means he is not to be resuscitated if BOTH his heart and lungs stop of natural causes from a terminal illness. The DNR status would be left on his records for the rest of his shortened life.

Steve didn't have a terminal illness on 06/24/15 which was three days after he had suffered a stroke and was scheduled to have stroke rehabilitation and therapy. X-rays indicated there was no further clotting/bleeding inside his brain. In other words, the stroke was over, the damage done leaving him temporarily unable to speak/swallow and paralyzed on his right side.

The fact that he passed out from fluid in his lungs was 100% caused by poor nursing/physician care and attention. They continued full feedings into his stomach and ignored 24 hours of increasing difficulty breathing which indicated he was drowning in the stomach fluids they were pushing in through his nose tube.

For anyone who has witnessed or read about strokes, his inability to swallow/speak and the one-sided paralysis is very common. Most people with left-sided stroke (affects the right side of the face and appendages) normally recover the ability to swallow first, followed by speech improvement next. With adequate physical therapy by professional therapists, the patient may even recover partial or full control over their paralyzed (one-sided) limbs.

On 06/26/15 an attempt was made to place Steve into palliative care and taken out of stroke rehabilitation/curative care. Steve wasn't asked if he was ready to die. His Brother refused to sign Steve into palliative care (hospice) when he met with Dr. Elizabeth McInerney who told him Steve's prognosis was grim.

However Dr. Elizabeth McInerney was able to convince brother Don Hatch that the DNR (Do Not Resuscitate) order needed to be signed in case Steve went unresponsive again. Don was told that was an indication that he was dying from the stroke and there was no reason to resuscitate him a second time. However, the DNR order only applies if cardiac/pulmonary arrest occurs (both heart and lungs have stopped). "Unresponsive" does not indicate heart and lungs have ceased.

Don Hatch signed the DNR at Mercy Medical Center but refused to sign Steve into palliative care where he would get no stroke therapy. So on 06/29/15 the safer PEG tube placement (Percutaneous Endoscopic Gastrotomy) was put in. The Nasogastric tube was removed the following day when the healing around the PEG tube allowed feedings and medications to be started directly into his stomach.

His pyloric sphincter muscle at the top of the stomach was no longer obstructed by the NG tube and could resume working to prevent stomach fluids from backing up into his lungs unless he was vomiting.

Subsequent vomiting will occur at Blackhawk Life Care Center in Lake View, Iowa the week ending on 07/16/15 (second aspiration) requiring Steve to be rushed to Loring Hospital, at Sac City Iowa for of the second aspiration incident. However, the second aspiration at Blackhawk Life Care was caused by excessive sedatives inducing ileus (vomiting).

By Marlys J. Waters
Blackhawk Life Care Center and Gentiva Hospice - Second Hospice Attempt

Steven Lee Hatch, age 66, had just been released from Mercy Medical Center in Sioux City on the evening or 07/07/15 after 17 days treatment for a stroke suffered 06/21/15. His stroke had stabilized according to brain scans so he was being released to Blackhawk Life Care Center to receive continuing stroke therapy/rehabilitation until he would be ready to return to his home He was paralyzed on his right side and unable to speak or to swallow. He was given nourishment through a PEG tube in his stomach.

Blackhawk Life Care Center in Lake View, Iowa wasn't qualified to accept a patient into their skilled care who would need specialized therapy/rehabilitation. However they also didn't want to turn away any patients as they were only operating at 53% occupancy. By admitting a stroke victim into skilled care who needed rehabilitation was only a temporary setback in nursing home finances in having to hire outside therapists. They should easily be able to get him into hospice so he could be downgraded to unskilled nursing care paid by the patient rather than by Medicare. After all, he was paralyzed on one side, couldn't talk or swallow, they could pretty much do as they pleased with him.

[Read the book I've republished "Dilemmas of Euthanasia" originally written in 1975 if you don't believe nursing homes and hospice work to get elderly residents out of Medicare and into hospice even if they don't have a terminal illness. MJW]

Blackhawk Life Care Center in Lake View made the decision to keep Steve at their facility by not allowing me to take him home. I had no legal right to take him home but that decision could have been solved by asking Steve and getting permission from the brother which wasn't done.

Blackhawk medical records show they were aware on the first full day 07/08/15 at Blackhawk Life Care Center that I was ready to take him home. In fact Marlys J. Waters would be the last person they would talk to about Steve's future, she could spoil their plans for months of unquestioned income. But first they had to get him into hospice and out of stroke rehabilitation.

Steve Hatch was admitted into skilled care along with the signed DNR (do not resuscitate) order that had been instigated by Dr. Shaheer Ahmed Siddiqui, a Hospitalist at Mercy Medical Center with referral and consultation by Dr. Elizabeth McInerney, Mercy Medical Center. The reason for the DNR was "grim prognosis for stroke recovery" as told to the clueless brother who had signed the DNR paper. But Don Hatch refused to sign Steve out of stroke therapy/rehabilitation and into Palliative/comfort care (hospice).

The DNR paper had no additional situations added to it. In the event of "cardio/pulmonary arrest" both his heart and lungs must stop before the caregivers could legally discontinue all care. If he aspirated again causing him to suffer from hypoxia (lack of oxygen to the brain) and he became unresponsive yet his heart was still beating, he was to be resuscitated.

The next day, 07/08/15 Blackhawk Life Care called in Gentiva Hospice to admit Steve into their program so he could be taken out of skilled care. Tracy Hinner, Director of nursing representing Blackhawk Life Care, Lake View had scheduled a meeting in the early afternoon with Heidi Schultes and Ann Lengeling representing Gentiva Hospice (now Kindred Hospice) out of their Carroll, Iowa office. Brother Don Hatch was not invited to that meeting nor was Marlys J. Waters.

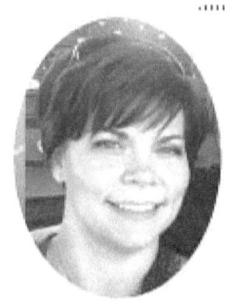

Ann Lengeling representing Gentiva Hospice
(now Kindred Hospice)
831 N Griffith Rd, Carroll, IA 51401
Phone: (712) 792-2191

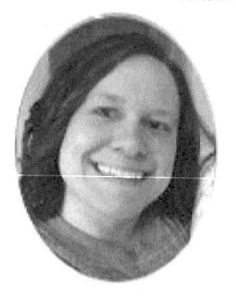

Heidi Pickhinke Schultes, representing Gentiva Hospice, (now Kindred Hospice)
831 N Griffith Rd, Carroll, IA 51401
Phone: (712) 792-2191

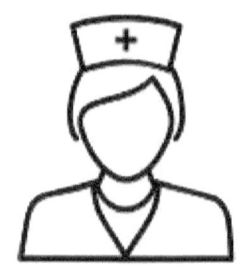

Tracy Hinners, R.N., Director of
Nursing/Operational/Manager
Blackhawk Life Care Center (Owned by
Capstone Management out of Des Moines)

However, that same afternoon on 07/08/15 I had just arrived at Blackhawk Life Care to visit Steve carrying a document from Steve's attorney, Erin McCullough, stating I had been declared Steve's legal Guardian/Conservator.

Ann Lengeling and Heidi Schultes representing Gentiva Hospice, (aka Kindred Hospice). Carroll, Iowa; and Tracy Hinner, Director of nursing representing Blackhawk Life Care, Lake View, invited me into a conference room and explained that Steve had indicated he wanted to die by pulling his PEG-tube (stomach feeding tube) loose, proof that he no longer wanted to live as a paralyzed man who is unable to speak or swallow.

They explained they could offer him palliative/comfort care until his death since that is what he obviously wanted. I knew that theory was a bunch of crap. Steve Hatch had a strong will to live and has a long history of pulling out tubes when he is ready to go home.

I listened while the three gals explained their training and background in assessing nursing home resident's needs and wishes. They reiterated on how important it is to make the patient's stay at the facility as calm and comfortable as possible. They also told me that in Gentiva Hospice, Steve would be given palliative medications to ease pain, depression, and restlessness.

Then I explained to Tracy, Ann, and Heidi that Steve's mind was fine. He could understand their words, but could only answer with yes/no. They could ask his permission for or against Hospice by using short sentences with non-technical jargon. It was up to Steve to make his own decision.

We went to his room where he was laying in bed with his head elevated. They took turns and asked the following questions:

1) Did he realize that without the feeding tube there was no way to feed him? "Yes"

2.) Did he want the feeding tube reinstalled? "Yes"

3.) Did he realize that having the stomach tube replaced meant he had to be taken by ambulance back to the hospital? "Yes"

Three times he answered "yes" in response to their questions while making eye contact with each gal. There was no hesitation, I was there, I saw his reaction. I could write a book about the number of times over the years that Steve had pulled out tubes, IVs, and other attachments when he had had enough medical care and was ready to go home. One I witnessed, the others he told me about.

Steve did not have a terminal illness. His stroke had stabilized and he had received a full week of therapy and rehabilitation at Mercy Medical Center with no additional complications after being resuscitated from caregiver negligence in allowing him to aspirate stomach fluids into his stomach resulting in hypoxia (lack of oxygen in the brain) with resulting unresponsive condition (he fainted). Steve did not want to die and he did not want to be put into a nursing home.

Legally only a person with a terminal illness can be admitted into hospice and they must request admittance themselves – no one can put a person into hospice without their permission, or if they are unconscious, it requires a court action before a judge by the family.

The fact that Gentiva Hospice was called AND showed up JUST because Steve might want to commit suicide rather than live life as a paralyzed man is proof that someone was planning to break a law by assisting him with what they thought was his wishes. Assisted Suicide is not legal in Iowa with or without a signed request to be admitted into Hospice. Suicide does not meet the requirement for "must have a terminal illness."

Note that this was one day after Steve Hatch had arrived at the nursing home in skilled care for stroke rehabilitation covered by Medicare for up to 90 days. However, if he was placed into hospice, Blackhawk Life Care Center could then charge Steve's room charge directly to him and hospice would be paid by Medicare. So Steve was worth more to Blackhawk Life Care as a hospice patient so they would no longer have to hire outside stroke therapists to treat him.

Hospice would then be paid by Medicare for their treatments, medications, and labor of physicians who prescribed palliative medications and nursing staff to administer all medications and supervise his care at Blackhawk. Hospice would also be paid for time spent counseling family.

At this point let's examine why Blackhawk wanted Steve put into hospice to die but did not want him to have the option to go back to his home with his Significant Other. Not once was Steve Hatch, Don Hatch nor Marlys Waters asked if Steve wanted to go home to die "from his terminal illness" (whatever that might have been.) Blackhawk and Gentiva Hospice had a temporarily silent and disabled man who was unable to fight back. This is why there was no discussion on giving Steve the option to return to his home. They wanted the money from his estate for room charges for as long as they wanted to keep him alive. Who would know he didn't have a terminal illness since the medications and coma-inducing sedatives were all given behind closed doors at the nursing home?

By Marlys J. Waters
Iowa State Hospice Rules 2015

1) "Hospice patient" or "patient" means a **diagnosed terminally ill person** with an anticipated life expectancy of six months or less, as certified by the attending physician, who, alone or in conjunction with a unit of care as defined in subsection 8, **has voluntarily requested** and received admission into the hospice program.
2) If the patient is unable to request admission, a family member may voluntarily request and receive admission on the patient's behalf. Hospice patient's family" means the immediate kin of the patient, including a spouse, parent, stepparent, brother, sister, stepbrother, stepsister, child, or stepchild. Additional relatives **or individuals with significant personal ties to the hospice patient may be included in the hospice patient's family.**
3) "Palliative care" means care directed at managing symptoms experienced by the hospice patient, as well as addressing related needs of the patient and family as they experience the stress of the dying process. The intent of palliative care is to enhance the quality of life for the hospice patient and family unit, and **is not treatment directed at cure of the terminal illness.**
4) "Unit of care" means the patient and the patient's family within a hospice program.

The hospice representatives and nursing home administrator believed it was perfectly legal to help a man commit suicide painlessly through hospice if he wanted to die rather than live as a paralyzed man who couldn't speak. I believe that the doctors and nurses did not want to bother themselves taking care of a man who could not swallow or talk. Do they even know that if he had been given adequate care he probably would have recovered most or all of his lost abilities? He was only 67 years old.

These steps of putting Steve Hatch into hospice illegally will eventually be accomplished by the medical staff and will directly cause his death. It is called "Involuntary Euthanasia" and it is illegal in Iowa.

Unfortunately for Blackhawk and Gentiva Hospice on 07/08/15, Steve indicated he was not ready to go into hospice in front of an important witness - his Significant Other (Marlys J. Waters). They would have to come up with a new plan. See the change in medication on 07/10/15 and what follows.

The next day I found out a judge decided to order a separate attorney to represent Steve at the Guardian/Conservator court appearance. Chuck Schulte was assigned with the court date scheduled for 08/10/15. That meant that Blackhawk needed to get Steve into hospice fast as they only had a month to get him out of skilled care and into unskilled care so they wouldn't need to pay for a month's stroke rehabilitation. They knew I wanted to take him home. Blackhawk Life Care needed a doctor to help them get Steve into hospice some other way. Read on, it just gets more weird.

In all 50 states, Involuntary Euthanasia is a crime. Depending on the circumstances, a person committing Euthanasia can be charged with a Class 2 felony, a Class 3 felony, a Class 4 felony or a Class A misdemeanor.

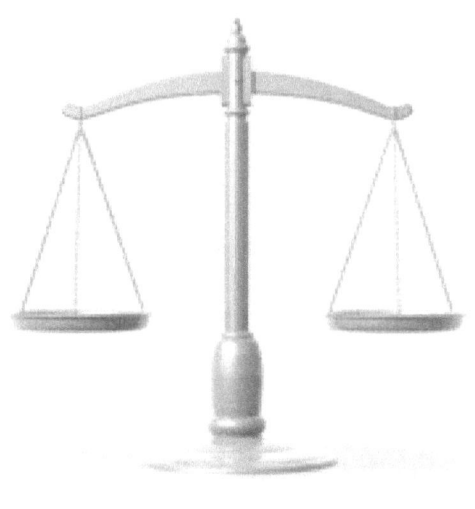

Patient Rights

By Marlys J. Waters

Blackhawk Hawk Life Care – Second Aspiration Incident

Steve Hatch had no terminal illness, the stroke had stabilized. He did not receive the stroke therapy and rehabilitation at Blackhawk Life Care Center in their skilled nursing care that he needed. He was given excessive medications that irritated his stomach and caused him to vomit. The inappropriate and dangerous opioid Lortab/Norco was administered for pain but he had no pain. I visited him every day and thought he was sleepy because of the therapist's rehabilitation exercises. I had no idea he was being given a very dangerous narcotic inappropriate for a partially paralyzed man whose heart and lungs could not function under a strong sedative.

1,001 Prescription Drugs ISBN1-890957-43-7   Prescription Drugs   29

ACETAMINOPHEN WITH HYDROCODONE BITARTRATE

Brand: Anexsia   Co-Gesic
        Hydrocet   Lorcet HD
        (Lortab)   Vicodin
        Vicodin ES Vicodin HP

This drug combines acetaminophen with a narcotic painkiller very similar to codeine and is used to relieve pain.

How to take this drug:
- Never take more medicine than you are prescribed.

Possible side effects:
Dizziness   Drowsiness
(Nausea)   Constipation
Mood changes   Mental clouding
Difficulty urinating Slow or irregular breathing

Possible interactions:
- If you take this drug along with alcohol or tranquilizers, antihistamines, or muscle relaxants, the combination may dangerously depress your nervous system.

Other important information:
- Hydrocodone suppresses the cough reflex, so people with lung disease should take this drug with caution.
- Use this drug with caution if you have a head injury, as it may increase fluid pressure on the brain.
- Older people and people with liver or kidney damage, an underactive thyroid, Addison's disease, or an enlarged prostate should take this drug with caution.
- You may become physically and psychologically dependent on this drug if you take high doses for long periods of time.

24 The Killing Field Known as Hospice

Steve Hatch was unable to swallow or to call for help. He was left laying in bed at Blackhawk Life Care for over 4 days starting on 07/13/15 as his lungs were again slowly filling up with his own vomit, a side effect of Lortab in combination with other medications. The Blackhawk Life Care medical records show an hourly mitt check where Steve was using the white protective cover over his left hand to try to clear his mouth of vomit, some days up to 8 continuous hours, an obvious unmonitored side effect of one (or more) medications that were ignored.

After Steve was having noticeable trouble breathing, he was taken to Loring Hospital by ambulance for treatment of aspiration pneumonia on the evening of 07/16/15. The strong narcotic Lortab/Norco which Dr. Marczewski had prescribed for use at Blackhawk Life Care Center to be used at their discretion every 6 hours for pain was suddenly stopped during his stay at Loring Hospital. Guess all his pain suddenly disappeared??? Or maybe there was NO pain in the first place???

I do not know who at Blackhawk Life Care Center asked Dr. Marczewski to prescribe a strong opioid for pain. Maybe it was Dr. Marczewski's idea? His name seems to come up a lot when there is a change of condition or care of Steve. You will see from the medication records that what happens next is just as ludicrous. Steve didn't have a chance to fight back once he was forced into hospice. Too many people were trying to get him out of skilled nursing care. Just pull the plug, who cares.

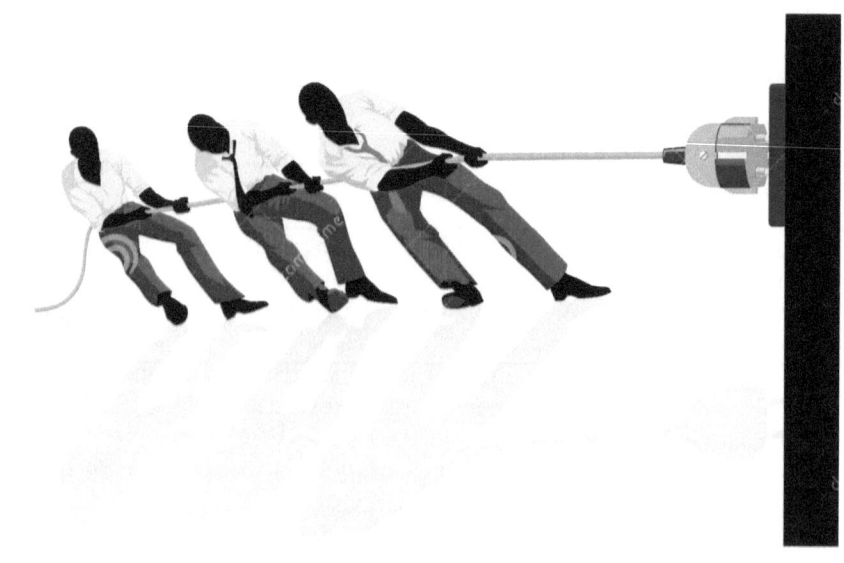

Loring Hospital Critical Care 07/16/15 – 07/20/15

Steve Hatch was taken by ambulance from Blackhawk Life Care Center on the evening of 07/16/15 after he was having great difficulty breathing. He had been vomiting for over four days and his lungs filled up with stomach fluids to the point of unconsciousness. (2nd time) The medication that caused the nausea was primarily Lortab, a very dangerous opioid prescribed by Dr. Marczewski to be used by the nurses at Blackhawk Life Care Center on Steve Hatch every 6 hours as needed for pain. The Lortab was started on 07/10/15 two days after Blackhawk Life Care Center failed to get Steve Hatch enrolled into hospice on 07/08/15 per his verbal refusal.

Dr. Leszak Marczewski had not examined Steve Hatch prior to submitting the prescription for Lortab. However, Dr. Marczewski became the attending physician when Steve Hatch was admitted to Loring on 07/16/15. There was NO Lortab or other dangerous opioid prescribed or administered at Loring Hospital. Looks like a cover-up for a medication that should not have been prescribed in the first place.

However, Dr. Marczewski was able to convince the nurses and other staff that he knew what he was doing. I visited Steve every day at Loring. I would check in at the Nurse's station to see if it was all right to visit him. One time a nurse made the comment that it would be better if the feedings and medications were stopped as there was no chance for recovery. She continued "He would not want to live LIKE THAT!"

I wanted to tell her there are some people who should not be allowed to live "STUPID" like her but I held my comment and said nothing.

The nurse obviously could see no reason to waste time treating a man who was paralyzed on one side and unable to swallow/speak. Because she made that comment at the nurse's station in front of a couple of other nurses and some visitors walking by meant that the nurses were just passing on the opinion of the attending physician Dr. Leszak Marczewski.

She must not know that a majority of stroke victims are in the same shape and a left sided stroke (affects the right side) are the easiest to cure with a better chance of recovery since they rarely affect the person's cognitive powers (the mind). A person with a good mind can live with proper care and continue to contribute to society.

Steven Hawking is in much worse shape than Steve Hatch and has not one chance of improving. He has spent years working as a scientist in a body that is unable to speak, move, or care for himself. Even in that state, his second wife continues to support and care for him just because he is a human being that gives joy just by living.

26 The Killing Field Known as Hospice

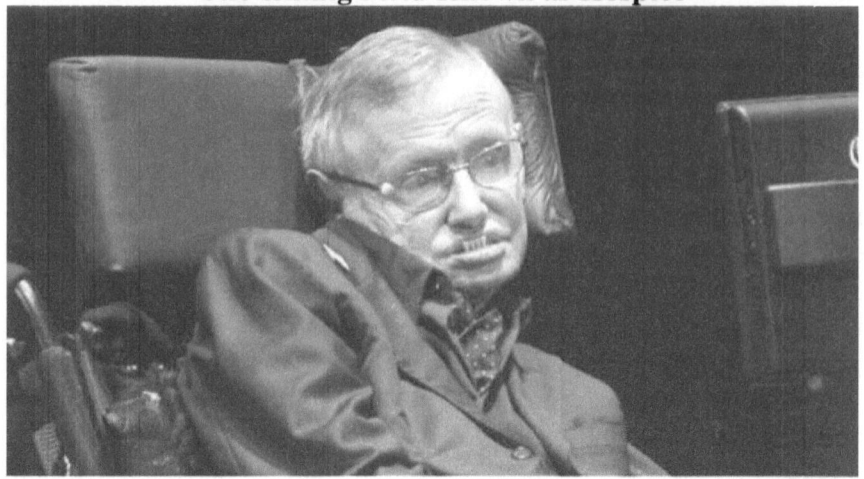

In 1963, Hawking contracted motor neurone disease and was given two years to live. Yet he went on to Cambridge to become a brilliant researcher and Professorial Fellow at Gonville and Caius College. From 1979 to 2009 he held the post of Lucasian Professor at Cambridge, the chair held by Isaac Newton in 1663.

Professor Hawking has over a dozen honorary degrees and was awarded the CBE in 1982. He is a fellow of the Royal Society and a Member of the US National Academy of Science. Stephen Hawking is regarded as one of the most brilliant theoretical physicists since Einstein. In January 2018 He is still alive and working daily.

My buddy Steve Hatch had an active and sometimes ornery mind with a great sense of humor. While his mind functioned differently due to a childhood skull fracture, he still was very smart in doing mechanical work on his antique tractors, riding lawn mowers, and automobiles. He also picked up how to operate and do computer searches without ever having prior training on a computer.

We sold black walnuts through ebay that he picked up each fall and cracked. He also bought things through ebay like a couple of C E Potter nut crackers made in the 1930's that were easiest to use on hard-shelled black walnuts. He'd wear one out every two years.

I ran a used book store and he enjoyed helping me sort books. He also helped me get a good start on collecting used music store inventory.

Steve Hatch had a good mind after the stroke. I was able to communicate with him just by watching his eyes and his facial expressions. If he wanted something like a pillow off the spare bed at the nursing home, he was able to tell me just by pointing with his un-paralyzed hand (which was enclosed in a white, padded mitt.)

He also looked in the direction of the stand by his bed indicating he needed his reading glasses when I was showing him pictures on my laptop of his garden, his geese and his barn cats that he hadn't seen for over a month. I had brought his reading glasses earlier to show him some birthday cards that came in the mail for his 67th birthday on 07/13/15 and he remembered the glasses were still in that stand.

I had told Steve two days after his stroke on 06/23/15 when he was in the stroke ward at Mercy Medical Center in Sioux City that I had made an offer to buy a handicapped accessible house in Nemaha that would simplify his recovery and mobility on wood floors using a wheelchair and a much larger bathroom. He knew what house I was talking about but he didn't say anything that day. Then on 07/28/15 after he had been in hospice for four days, he asked me if I had possession of the house yet.

All he needed to say was "houssss" "Houssss" twice and I replied "You want to know if I have possession of the house yet?" And he shook his head "yes". I explained that the offer had been accepted and I was just waiting for the paperwork to be made up. I also added that I couldn't take him home until a couple of weeks when I had a court date to request being awarded his legal guardian/conservator.

Steve seemed a little more content on that day. But unknown to me that was 07/28/15, the day he was put back on Lortab and started sleeping a lot during my subsequent visits. While he had been put into hospice, I wasn't worried because I knew he didn't have a terminal illness and that I could do more for his recovery if I could get him home and work with him along with the therapists through home-health care.

I could also cancel hospice after I became his guardian. What I didn't know is that he had been taken out of skilled nursing care which meant he was no longer receiving stroke rehabilitation. I thought he was sleeping more when I came for my daily 2-4 hour visits due to his therapy exercises. I did not know about any dangerous narcotics/opioids until after his death when I used my "co-administrator of his estate" status to request all his medical records. I believe brother Don Hatch also wanted the best for his brother and had given Steve's attorney permission to grant me co-administrator of Steve's estate plus Guardian/Conservator status.

I also had no idea that the aspiration pneumonia that caused him to be hospitalized was caused by Lortab which induced vomiting and filled his lungs. I had taken care of my mother as she was dying of pancreatic cancer and who I fed through a PEG-tube just like Steve had. I only had trouble with her aspirating the liquids on her final four days. The hospice workers that came to the house every day for an hour said that she must have water for hydration but the nutrient solution might be harder for her to digest so they recommended diluting the feeding nutrient 50/50 with water which resulted in fewer residue between feedings and less trouble breathing during her last days.

The hospice workers in 2002 did not force mother to take any sedatives if she didn't need them. They would ask her during their daily visit if she had any pain. She always replied that she did not. She was just slowly starving to death because she could no longer digest any foods. I was so glad that I had moved back to my hometown to be able to take care of both of my parents in their final years.

My father had a heart attack at age 91 and died sitting upright in a chair. Some deaths are easy, cancer like my mother had is always difficult.

Then there are the deaths that are caused by involuntary euthanasia like Steve Hatch. This experience just shows how barbaric our culture is that allows a man to be murdered in public just because he had suffered a stroke.

The doctors didn't have to care for him any longer, all they had to do was let me take him home and care for him. I'm sure he would have lived a lot longer under my care. I had worked with him for 12 years to keep him healthy and checked his medications for safety and being taken on schedule.

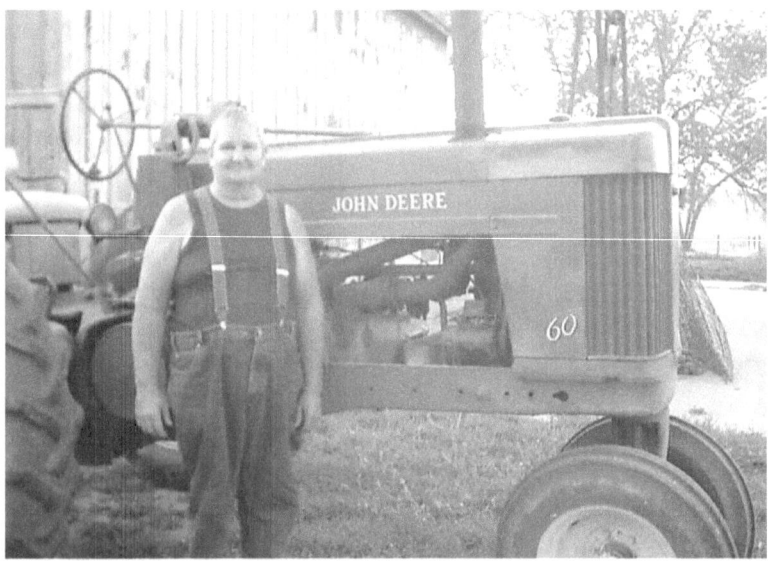

Steve Hatch and one of his many antique tractors.

By Marlys J. Waters
About Steve's Fractured Skull at age 6 on May 2, 1955

Steve Hatch was nearing the end of first grade at the Early, Iowa school at the age of 6 when he suffered a fractured skull. A classmate, Tim Ellinger, pushed him over a railing by the old Early school gym on May 2, 1955. He landed on his head on cement a floor below near the stairwell by the gymnasium. He had blood coming out of his eyes, ears, nose and mouth.

Steve was taken to Loring Hospital in Sac City, Iowa where he was in a coma for four days and not expected to live. However he survived and was released from the hospital on May 13, eleven days later but was unable to speak.

In October of 1955 he was sent to Iowa City accompanied by his mother for a month of speech therapy to regain his ability to speak. Steve was able to return to school with the same classmates later in the fall of 1955.

Eventually he was kept back a grade and was supposed to graduate with the class of 1967. His thinking was a bit off yet he was NOT dumb. He was not given remedial training, summer classes, nor a tutor as assistance for his disability. The Early school originally paid for his hospital bills, nothing else.

Steve Hatch was asked to leave school and not return after he had turned 16. Nemaha and Early had combined by then and the Crestland School principal, William Hall, told him there was no reason for him to come to school as he was not going to graduate anyway.

Without coming close to getting a high school diploma, Steve Hatch did not qualify for any higher education. Even getting hired in cushy jobs was hard without a high school diploma. So he farmed with his father until his parents retired from farming, then he took whatever jobs he could get and worked hard to keep them, never taking sick days or even vacation time.

Steve Hatch's final job ruined his lungs diesel truck exhaust fumes. I worked at BilMar Turkey processing plant in Storm Lake, Iowa for two years and I quit when I developed a cough I couldn't get rid of and also would get migraine aura/headaches during the winter months. I still get migraine auras when I'm around automotive exhaust fumes and which had caused my lung/head problems when I worked at BilMar.

Steve Hatch was working at BilMar at the same time I was only he worked the night shift for 10 years. During that time Steve developed COPD (emphysema) from the diesel truck fumes in the unloading area which ruined his lungs. So at the age of 54 his working days were over and he was forced to go on Social Security Disability. He followed doctor's orders as best he could but some medications interacted with others and those that helped his breathing may have ruined his heart value (aortic stenosis) and contributed to mild diabetes which was controlled with limiting sugar intake, exercise, and a couple of pills per day.

So why am I giving you Steve's medical history? Because the stroke was an indirect reaction to his other medical disorders. One lady cardiologist got mad at him for not getting his heart operated on. She didn't care that he was suffering from GI bleeding that had led to multiple hospitalizations between 2013-2014. He required many pints of blood transfusions during that year, some as an outpatient, others with overnight stays in the hospital.

How can a person be expected to go to Rochester for a heart operation when the local doctors can't even figure out why he is losing so much blood? I place the fact that he had a stroke being caused by the pulmonary specialist, the cardiologist, and the general practitioner not working together. So now Steve is completely (possibly only temporarily) disabled from a stroke and the whole medical profession chalks him off as not worth saving, as having no value as a human being.

In the spring of 2015 Steve Hatch was feeling better than he had felt in years. He was working too hard but couldn't be slowed down. I'm sure he would have worked just as hard following recommended instructions in stroke therapy. Between the two of us, we might have even invented some new equipment to help other people with strokes, or at least written a book about his recovery and suggestions to help others.

Instead, the medical people didn't think his life was worth saving, that he had nothing further left to justify his existence. He was forced into hospice without a terminal illness and without his permission. Hospice is not closely monitored as it is used for elderly, disabled people near death. There are no public officials monitoring what goes on in hospice. If the people are in pain, the nurses are allowed to use as many pain killers as necessary, even if they accidentally cause the person's heart and lungs to stop.

Steve Hatch was not dying of anything. His COPD, heart disorder, paralyzed right side, inability to speak, diabetes, were all stable. People recovering from stokes usually improve. The only ones that don't are those who are euthanized because no one wants to take care of them. Steve had someone who wanted to take care of him.

This is why Steve Hatch's death has to be treated as "involuntary Euthanasia" which is illegal and punishable in Iowa as a felony. He was purposefully put into hospice (illegally) and his heart and lungs were slowed down with Lortab (gasping for air) followed by Morphine (to stop his heart and lungs.)

Blackhawk Life Care Center – Narcotics/Opioids 07/07/15 – 07/16/15

The following chart I put together only shows the Lortab that I suspect caused him to be vomiting which filled his lungs. It includes the dates/times of stomach residue when the liquid feedings were not being digested completely. The hourly mitt check "code 8" is the only indication I have proving that he was vomiting which caused his lungs to fill with fluid. There are also code 2 (drug refused) and 5 (see progress notes) which I do not know what they mean.

This chart ends when Steve is taken by ambulance to Loring Hospital to be treated the second time for aspiration pneumonia.

	Lortab/Stomach Residue Comparison 7/7/2015 - 7/16/15	
	Med	Given by/Reaction
07/08/15 2130	Check residual prioir to feeding 6xday	residual 11
07/08/15 2200	Enteral Feed order Glucerna 1.0 320cc 6xday	**Code 8 Vomiting**
07/08/15 2359	Enteral Feed order Glucerna 1.0 320cc 6xday	**Code 5 see progress notes**
07/09/15 0000	Inject 0.1 cc Tubersol Solution for testing	**WR code 8 vomiting**
07/09/15 0130	Check residual prioir to feeding 6xday	residual 5
07/09/15 0200	Enteral Feed order Glucerna 1.0 320cc 6xday	**Code 5 see progress notes**
07/09/15 0530	Check residual prioir to feeding 6xday	residual 60
07/09/15 0600	Insulin Detemir Solution 100 Unit/ML re: DIAB	60 unit once daily **code 5 Hold**
07/09/15 1000	Pulmicort Suspension 0.5 MG/2ML Budesonide 1 dose inhaled 2xday	By TD **Code 8 vomiting, Hold**
07/09/15 1330	Check residual prioir to feeding 6xday	residual 10
07/09/15 2130	Check residual prioir to feeding 6xday	residual 10

07/10/15 0130	Check residual prioir to feeding 6xday	**residual 10**
07/10/15 0530	Check residual prioir to feeding 6xday	**residual 15**
07/10/15 0930	Check residual prioir to feeding 6xday	**residual 4**
07/10/15 1330	Check residual prioir to feeding 6xday	**residual 5**
07/10/15 1730	Check residual prioir to feeding 6xday	**residual 5**
07/10/15 1900	**Lortab Tab 5-325 MG Hydrocodone-Acetaminophen via PEG-tube prn 6 hrs pain**	By CK Effective
07/11/15 0125	**Lortab Tab 5-325 MG Hydrocodone-Acetaminophen via PEG-tube prn 6 hrs pain**	By TB Effective
07/11/15 1330	Check residual prioir to feeding 6xday	**residual 4**
07/11/15 1620	**Lortab Tab 5-325 MG Hydrocodone-Acetaminophen via PEG-tube prn 6 hrs pain**	By WR Effective
07/11/15 1730	Check residual prioir to feeding 6xday	**residual 5**
07/12/15 0200	Left hand safety mitt checked hourly (PEG-tube)	By TB **Code 5 see progress notes**
07/12/15 0300	Left hand safety mitt checked hourly (PEG-tube)	By TB **Code 5 see progress notes**
07/12/15 0400	Left hand safety mitt checked hourly (PEG-tube)	By TB **Code 5 see progress notes**
07/12/15 0500	Left hand safety mitt checked hourly (PEG-tube)	By TB **Code 5 see progress notes**
07/12/15 0600	Left hand safety mitt checked hourly (PEG-tube)	By TB **Code 5 see progress notes**

07/12/15 0700	Left hand safety mitt checked hourly (PEG-tube)	By TB **Code 5 see progress notes**
07/12/15 0800	Left hand safety mitt checked hourly (PEG-tube)	By KS **Code 5 see progress notes**
07/12/15 0900	Left hand safety mitt checked hourly (PEG-tube)	By TB **+Code 5 see progress notes**
07/12/15 1000	Left hand safety mitt checked hourly (PEG-tube)	By KS **Code 5 see progress notes**
07/12/15 1100	Left hand safety mitt checked hourly (PEG-tube)	By KS **Code 8 nausea/vomit**
07/12/15 1200	Left hand safety mitt checked hourly (PEG-tube)	By KS **Code 8 nausea/vomit**
07/12/15 1300	Left hand safety mitt checked hourly (PEG-tube)	By KS **Code 8 nausea/vomit**
07/12/15 1330	Check residual prioir to feeding 6xday	**residual 30**
07/12/15 1400	Left hand safety mitt checked hourly (PEG-tube)	By KS **Code 8 nausea/vomit**
07/12/15 1546	**Lortab Tab 5-325 MG Hydrocodone-Acetaminophen via PEG-tube prn 6 hrs pain**	By WR Effective
07/12/15 1730	Check residual prioir to feeding 6xday	**residual 10**
07/13/15 0040	**Lortab Tab 5-325 MG Hydrocodone-Acetaminophen via PEG-tube prn 6 hrs pain**	By TB Effective
07/13/15 0200	Left hand safety mitt checked hourly (PEG-tube)	By TB **Code 5 see progress notes**
07/13/15 0300	Left hand safety mitt checked hourly (PEG-tube)	By TB **Code 5 see progress notes**
07/13/15 0400	Left hand safety mitt checked hourly (PEG-tube)	By TB **Code 5 see progress notes**

The Killing Field Known as Hospice

Date/Time	Action	Result
07/13/15 0500	Left hand safety mitt checked hourly (PEG-tube)	By TB **Code 5 see prog notes**
07/13/15 0530	Check residual prioir to feeding 6xday	**residual 5**
07/13/15 0600	Left hand safety mitt checked hourly (PEG-tube)	**Code 5 see progress notes**
07/13/15 0600	Singulair Tablet (Montelukast Sodium) 10 MG prevent sob	one time a day PEG-t
07/13/15 0700	Left hand safety mitt checked hourly (PEG-tube)	By KS **Code 5 see progress notes**
07/13/15 0800	Left hand safety mitt checked hourly (PEG-tube)	By KS **Code 5 see progress notes**
07/13/15 0900	Left hand safety mitt checked hourly (PEG-tube)	By KS **Code 5 see progress notes**
07/13/15 1000	Left hand safety mitt checked hourly (PEG-tube)	By KS **Code 5 see progress notes**
07/13/15 1500	Left hand safety mitt checked hourly (PEG-tube)	By JR **Code 2 drug refused**
07/13/15 1600	Left hand safety mitt checked hourly (PEG-tube)	By JR **Code 2 drug refused**
07/13/15 1700	Left hand safety mitt checked hourly (PEG-tube)	By JR **Code 2 drug refused**
07/13/15 1730	Check residual prioir to feeding 6xday	**residual 5**
07/13/15 1800	Left hand safety mitt checked hourly (PEG-tube)	By JR **Code 2 drug refused**
07/13/15 1900	**Lortab Tab 5-325 MG Hydrocodone-Acetaminophen via PEG-tube prn 6 hrs pain**	By TB Effective
07/13/15 2100	Left hand safety mitt checked hourly (PEG-tube)	By WR **Code 8 nausea/vomit**
07/13/15 2200	Left hand safety mitt checked hourly (PEG-tube)	By WR **Code 8 nausea/vomit**

07/13/15 2300	Left hand safety mitt checked hourly (PEG-tube)	By WR **Code 8 nausea/vomit**
07/14/15 0000	Left hand safety mitt checked hourly (PEG-tube)	By WR **Code 8 nausea/vomit**
07/14/15 0100	Left hand safety mitt checked hourly (PEG-tube)	By WR **Code 8 nausea/vomit**
07/14/15 0130	**Lortab Tab 5-325 MG Hydrocodone-Acetaminophen via PEG-tube prn 6 hrs pain**	By WR Effective
07/14/15 0200	Left hand safety mitt checked hourly (PEG-tube)	By WR **Code 8 nausea/vomit**
07/14/15 0300	Left hand safety mitt checked hourly (PEG-tube)	By WR **Code 8 nausea/vomit**
07/14/15 0400	Left hand safety mitt checked hourly (PEG-tube)	By WR **Code 8 nausea/vomit**
07/14/15 0500	Left hand safety mitt checked hourly (PEG-tube)	By WR **Code 8 nausea/vomit**
07/14/15 0600	Left hand safety mitt checked hourly (PEG-tube)	By WR **Code 8 nausea/vomit**
07/14/15 0700	Left hand safety mitt checked hourly (PEG-tube)	By KS **Code 5 see progress notes**
07/14/15 0800	Left hand safety mitt checked hourly (PEG-tube)	By KS **Code 5 see progress notes**
07/14/15 0900	Left hand safety mitt checked hourly (PEG-tube)	By KS **Code 5 see progress notes**
07/14/15 0930	Check residual prioir to feeding 6xday	**residual 5**
07/14/15 1000	Left hand safety mitt checked hourly (PEG-tube)	By KS **Code 5 see progress notes**
07/14/15 1000	Left hand safety mitt checked hourly (PEG-tube)	By KS **Code 5 see progress notes**
07/14/15 1100	Left hand safety mitt checked hourly (PEG-tube)	By KS **Code 5 see progress notes**

Date/Time	Action	Notes
07/14/15 1200	Left hand safety mitt checked hourly (PEG-tube)	By KS **Code 5** see progress notes
07/14/15 1200	Left hand safety mitt checked hourly (PEG-tube)	By KS **Code 5** see progress notes
07/14/15 1200	Left hand safety mitt checked hourly (PEG-tube)	By KS **Code 5** see progress notes
07/14/15 1400	Left hand safety mitt checked hourly (PEG-tube)	By KS **Code 5** see progress notes
07/15/15 0600	Left hand safety mitt checked hourly (PEG-tube)	By TB **Code 8 nausea/vomit**
07/15/15 0600	Singulair Tablet (Montelukast Sodium) 10 MG prevent sob	one time a day PEG-t
07/15/15 0700	Left hand safety mitt checked hourly (PEG-tube)	By KS **Code 5** see progress notes
07/15/15 0800	Left hand safety mitt checked hourly (PEG-tube)	By KS **Code 5** see progress notes
07/15/15 0900	Left hand safety mitt checked hourly (PEG-tube)	By KS **Code 5** see progress notes
07/15/15 1100	Left hand safety mitt checked hourly (PEG-tube)	By KS **Code 5** see progress notes
07/15/15 1300	Left hand safety mitt checked hourly (PEG-tube)	By KS **Code 5** see progress notes
07/15/15 1400	Left hand safety mitt checked hourly (PEG-tube)	By KS **Code 5** see progress notes
07/15/15 1700	Left hand safety mitt checked hourly (PEG-tube)	By WR **Code 8 nausea/vomit**
07/15/15 1800	Left hand safety mitt checked hourly (PEG-tube)	By WR **Code 8 nausea/vomit**
07/15/15 1900	Left hand safety mitt checked hourly (PEG-tube)	By WR **Code 8 nausea/vomit**

07/15/15 2000	Left hand safety mitt checked hourly (PEG-tube)	By WR **Code 8 nausea/vomit**
07/15/15 2100	Left hand safety mitt checked hourly (PEG-tube)	**Code 8 nausea/vomit**
07/15/15 2200	Left hand safety mitt checked hourly (PEG-tube)	**Code 8 nausea/vomit**
07/15/15 2300	Left hand safety mitt checked hourly (PEG-tube)	**Code 8 nausea/vomit**
07/16/15 0000	Left hand safety mitt checked hourly (PEG-tube)	By WR **Code 8 nausea/vomit**
07/16/15 0037	**Lortab Tab 5-325 MG Hydrocodone-Acetaminophen via PEG-tube prn 6 hrs pain**	By WR Effective
07/16/15 0100	Left hand safety mitt checked hourly (PEG-tube)	By WR **Code 8 nausea/vomit**
07/16/15 0130	Check residual prior to feeding if over 100 hold	6 times a day 5
07/16/15 0200	Left hand safety mitt checked hourly (PEG-tube)	By WR **Code 8 nausea/vomit**
07/16/15 0300	Left hand safety mitt checked hourly (PEG-tube)	By WR **Code 8 nausea/vomit**
07/16/15 0400	Left hand safety mitt checked hourly (PEG-tube)	By WR **Code 8 nausea/vomit**
07/16/15 0500	Left hand safety mitt checked hourly (PEG-tube)	By WR **Code 8 nausea/vomit**
07/16/15 0530	Check residual prior to feeding if over 100 hold	6 times a day 15
07/16/15 0600	Left hand safety mitt checked hourly (PEG-tube)	By WR **Code 8 nausea/vomit**
07/16/15 0700	Left hand safety mitt checked hourly (PEG-tube)	By JR **Code 5 see progress notes**
07/16/15 0800	Left hand safety mitt checked hourly (PEG-tube)	By JR **Code 5 see progress notes**

07/16/15 0834	**Lortab Tab 5-325 MG Hydrocodone-Acetaminophen via PEG-tube prn 6 hrs pain**	By WR Effective
07/16/15 0900	Left hand safety mitt checked hourly (PEG-tube)	By JR **Code 5 see progress notes**
07/16/15 0930	Check residual prior to feeding if over 100 hold	6 times a day 4
07/16/15 1000	Left hand safety mitt checked hourly (PEG-tube)	By JR **Code 5 see progress notes**
07/16/15 1100	Left hand safety mitt checked hourly (PEG-tube)	By JR **Code 5 see progress notes**
07/16/15 1200	Left hand safety mitt checked hourly (PEG-tube)	By JR **Code 5 see progress notes**
07/16/15 1300	Left hand safety mitt checked hourly (PEG-tube)	By JR **Code 5 see progress notes**
07/16/15 1330	Check residual prioir to feeding 6xday	**residual 8**
07/16/15 1330	Check residual prioir to feeding 6xday	**residual 25**
07/16/15 1400	Left hand safety mitt checked hourly (PEG-tube)	By JR **Code 5 see progress notes**
07/16/15 1500	Left hand safety mitt checked hourly (PEG-tube)	By JR **Code 5 see progress notes**
07/16/15 1700	Left hand safety mitt checked hourly (PEG-tube)	By CK **Code 8 nausea/vomit**
07/16/15 1800	Left hand safety mitt checked hourly (PEG-tube)	By CK **Code 8 nausea/vomit**
07/16/15 1900	Left hand safety mitt checked hourly (PEG-tube)	By CK **Code 8 nausea/vomit**

By Marlys J. Waters

Steve Hatch Was Successfully Treated at Loring Hospital For Aspiration Pneumonia

Within four days Steve's lungs were clear of fluid, he was conscious and comfortable. On 07/20/15 he was processed for release to go back to Blackhawk Life Care Center to resume skilled nursing care with stroke rehabilitation.

However Blackhawk didn't want him back in skilled care paid by Medicare where they would be required to give him stroke rehabilitation. So Steve didn't leave the hospital and was readmitted into curative care at Loring.

So the attending physician Dr. Leszak Marczewski called in the brother and told him the prognosis for Steve's recovery was not good and that he should be placed into Hospice. Brother Don Hatch said he would consider it and left.

Dr. Marczewski then ordered four more days of excessive steroids/sedatives/nebulizer treatments and other unneeded and dangerous medications – but no narcotics. The result was that within four additional days Steve's awareness had declined to the point that Dr. Marczewski noted on the 07/24/15 discharge records that he was "comatose".

Then he had ordered a public van with a wheelchair lift. Steve was placed (comatose ? and paralyzed ?) sitting upright in a wheelchair on a hot July day without external oxygen and rolled out to the public van driven by a bus driver (not a trained medical ambulance personnel).

By the time the van arrived 30 minutes later at Blackhawk Life Care Center in Lake View, Iowa, Steve had fainted due to lack of oxygen during the public van ride on the sweltering hot July day. He fainted from lack of oxygen to the brain (hypoxia).

Blackhawk Life Care refused to accept him as unconscious unless they could use the DNR order to let him lay in bed until his death. Steve Hatch was not in hospice at that time. They called me at home to see if it was all right to honor the DNR order (do not resuscitate). I explained that they needed to check his respiration and his heart beat. If his heart was still beating and he was still breathing, then the DNR did not apply. Not all doctors or nurses understood the "exceptions" on Steve's DNR document had NOT been checked which would have allowed additional reasons for not resuscitating him even if his heart was still beating.

So Blackhawk called an ambulance manned by EMTs with oxygen and returned Steve back to Loring Hospital Emergency Room with oxygen, air-conditioning and reclining with his head elevated on the stretcher rather than sitting up with his chin on his chest in a wheelchair in a public transport van. Steve was conscious and alert by the time the ambulance got him back to the ER at Loring hospital.

Steve was readmitted by a different doctor less than two hours after Dr. Marczewski (who had since disappeared.) had discharged Steve from Loring and ordered the van ride. Dr. Hugh Leigh had never seen Steve Hatch before. He examined Steve in the emergency room. Tests were run, Steve was alert (eyes open, making eye contact, answering questions with yes/no.)

Steve was diagnosed and treated for hypoxia (lack of oxygen to the brain). Dr. Leigh did not know about the inappropriate van ride. Then Dr. Hugh Leigh noticed on the recent medical records that "family was considering hospice" so someone went ahead and called in the brother, hospice representatives and helped admit Steve Hatch into hospice without a terminal illness and .without his permission (he was conscious when the papers were signed).

Steve had verbally declined admittance into hospice on July 8, 2015 to Heidi Pickhinke Schultus, Tracy Hinner, and Ann Lengeling. Yet on July 24, 2015 Heidi Pickhinke Schultus still representing Gentia Hispice, signed the papers anyway to admit Steve into hospice along with Dr. Michael Slattery as the Hospice Physician who handled the referral by telephone, and by Dr. Hugh Leigh, the attending physician at Loring. This time Steve was not asked if he was ready for hospice. Heidi Schultus must have forgotten that Steve Hatch had said NO to Hospice just sixteen days earlier.

Within a couple of hours Steve was taken by ambulance back to Blackhawk Life Care Center who would now accept him into their **UN-SKILLED** care without stroke therapy/rehabilitation necessary. Steve was no longer covered by Medicare for Blackhawk room charges which would be billed to him personally.

Hospice would now be paid by Medicare for fulltime nursing care until Steve dies of his terminal illness. Wait a minute; **Steve didn't have a terminal illness!** A stroke is not a terminal illness. Aspiration pneumonia caused by nausea from opioids which caused vomit to back up into his lungs is not a terminal illness. Subjecting him to 4 days of excessive and unneeded medications at Loring Hospital (no narcotics this time), then diagnose him as comatose and give him a ride sitting up in a wheelchair in a public transport van on a hot summer day without oxygen causing hypoxia is not a terminal illness. I would like to know what terminal illness he was supposedly dying from?

It appeared to me Steve Hatch was having trouble staying alive from people who wanted him dead, not from any illness.

Loring Hospital - Excessive Meds Over Extra Four Days

These excessive medications between 7/20/15 – 7/24/15 were given for no valid reason as Steve's vitals were stable and his lungs were clear on 07/20/15 when Steve was supposed to be released from Loring..

It appears Dr. Leszak Marczewski was trying to get Steve Hatch's health to decline so he could convince the brother that Steve needed to be placed into Hospice (third attempt to convince the brother). Blackhawk Life Care Center had did not want Steve returned into their skilled nursing care, and would only accept him if he was in hospice so they would no longer need to give him stroke rehabilitation.

The medications given between 07/20 – 07/24 where ones Steve had been prescribed in past years but had not needed them recently. The reaction between the **Corticosteroids** were counteracting with his diabetes causing rise in blood sugar requiring excessive insulin (see duel signoffs by the nurses) who were unable to correct the high blood-sugar. On 7/20/15 Steve's health was stable. By 7/24/15 after these excessive medications, his psychic had declined and he fainted. YOU figure out the motive.

	Monday July 20, 2015		
07/20/15 0041	Furosemide (LASIX) intravenous	40 mg intravenous	Emily J Lange RN
07/20/15 0105	Glucerna 1.0 CAL LIQD every 4 hours	320 mL PEG Tube	**HELD, fluid overload, SOB, LASIX given**
07/20/15 0400	Albuterol (PROVENTIL) nebulizer	2.5 mg	Emily J Lange RN
07/20/15 0535	Glucerna 1.0 CAL LIQD every 4 hours	320 mL PEG Tube	Emily J Lange RN
07/20/15 0758	**Budesonide (PULMICORT) nebulizer 2 daily**	**Corticosteroid** .5 mg	Phillip R. Glenn, RRT
07/20/15 0844	Ciprofloxacin in D5W IV 2 times per day	200 mL/hr / 60 min	Julia M Box, RN
07/20/15 0844	Diltiazem (CARDIZEM) tablet 4 times daily	30 mg per G Tube	Julia M Box, RN
07/20/15 0844	Montelukast (SINGULAIR tablet daily	10 mg per G Tube	Julia M Box, RN

The Killing Field Known as Hospice

Date/Time	Medication	Dose	Administered By
07/20/15 0844	Pantoprazole (PROTONIX) injection	40 mg intravenous	Julia M Box, RN
07/20/15 0844	**Prednisone (DELTASONE) tablet**	Corticosteroid 5 mg per G tube daily	Julia M Box, RN
07/20/15 0907	Glucerna 1.0 CAL LIQD every 4 hours	320 mL PEG Tube	Julia M Box, RN
07/20/15 1001	Furosemide (LASIX) intravenous	40 mg intravenous	Julia M Box, RN
07/20/15 1002	CefTRIAXone (ROCEPHIN) IVPB every 12 hours	100 mL/hr / 30 min.	Julia M Box, RN
07/20/15 1145	Diltiazem (CARDIZEM) tablet 4 times daily	30 mg per G Tube	Jill S Vonahn, RN
07/20/15 1416	Glucerna 1.0 CAL LIQD every 4 hours	320 mL PEG Tube	Jill S Vonahn, RN
07/20/15 1632	Furosemide (LASIX) intravenous	20 mg slow IV - 2 min.	Julia M Box, RN
07/20/15 1710	Diltiazem (CARDIZEM) tablet 4 times daily	30 mg per G Tube	Julia M Box, RN
07/20/15 1710	Glucerna 1.0 CAL LIQD every 4 hours	320 mL PEG Tube	Julia M Box, RN
07/20/15 1821	**Budesonide (PULMICORT) nebulizer 2 daily**	Corticosteroid .5 mg	Phillip R Glenn, RRT
07/20/15 1823	Albuterol (PROVENTIL) nebulizer	2.5 mg	Phillip R Glenn, RRT
07/20/15 2028	Diltiazem (CARDIZEM) tablet 4 times daily	30 mg per G Tube	Sara M Bell RN
07/20/15 2110	Ciprofloxacin in D5W IV 2 times per day	200 mL/hr / 60 min	Sara M Bell RN
07/20/15 2110	Insulin detemir (LEVEMIR FLEXPEN)subcutaneous	55 units, **dual signoff**	Amanda L Hedberg, Amanda J Nees
07/20/15 2154	Glucerna 1.0 CAL LIQD every 4 hours	320 mL PEG Tube	Emily J Lange RN

Date/Time	Medication	Dose	Nurse
07/20/15 2201	Insulin Aspart (NOVOLOG FLEXPEN) injection	5 units **dual signoff**	Sara M Bell RN & Emily Lange
07/20/15 2259	CefTRIAXone (ROCEPHIN) IVPB every 12 hours	100 mL/hr / 30 min.	Sara M Bell RN

Tuesday July 21, 2015

Date/Time	Medication	Dose	Nurse
07/21/15 0104	Albuterol (PROVENTIL) nebulizer	2.5 mg	Sara M Bell RN
07/21/15 0142	**MethylPREDISolone sodium succinate injection**	**Corticosteroid 40 mg IV 3-5 min**	Sara M Bell RN
07/21/15 0143	Furosemide (LASIX) intravenous	40 mg slow IV - 2 min.	Sara M Bell RN
07/21/15 0159	Glucerna 1.0 CAL LIQD every 4 hours	320 mL PEG Tube	**HELD, fluid overload**
07/21/15 0618	Glucerna 1.0 CAL LIQD every 4 hours	320 mL PEG Tube	Sara M Bell RN
07/21/15 0639	Insulin Aspart (NOVOLOG FLEXPEN) injection	5 units **dual signoff BS 343**	Sara M Bell RN & Emily Lange
07/21/15 0805	Albuterol (PROVENTIL) nebulizer	2.5 mg	Phillip R Glenn, RRT
07/21/15 0805	**Budesonide (PULMICORT) nebulizer 2 daily**	**Corticosteroid** .5 mg	Phillip R Glenn, RRT
07/21/15 0935	Diltiazem (CARDIZEM) tablet 4 times daily	30 mg per G Tube	Molly J Sporrer, RN
07/21/15 0935	Montelukast (SINGULAIR tablet daily	10 mg per G Tube	Molly J Sporrer, RN
07/21/15 0935	**Prednisone (DELTASONE) tablet**	**Corticosteroid** 5 mg per G tube daily	Molly J Sporrer, RN
07/21/15 0936	Ciprofloxacin in D5W IV 2 times per day	200 mL/hr / 60 min	Molly J Sporrer, RN
07/21/15 0936	Furosemide (LASIX) intravenous	20 mg slow IV - 2 min.	Molly J Sporrer, RN

Date/Time	Medication	Dose	Administered By
07/21/15 0936	Pantoprazole (PROTONIX) injection	40 mg intravenous	Molly J Sporrer, RN
07/21/15 1053	CefTRIAXone (ROCEPHIN) IVPB every 12 hours	100 mL/hr / 30 min.	Karla J Grote, RN
07/21/15 1054	Glucerna 1.0 CAL LIQD every 4 hours	320 mL PEG Tube	Karla J Grote, RN
07/21/15 1122	Insulin Aspart (NOVOLOG FLEXPEN) injection	7 units **dual signoff** Karla J Grote/Julia M Box	**Dr. Marczewski, one order 7 units, glucose 557**
07/21/15 1259	Diltiazem (CARDIZEM) tablet 4 times daily	30 mg per G Tube	Karla J Grote, RN
07/21/15 1401	Glucerna 1.0 CAL LIQD every 4 hours	320 mL PEG Tube	Karla J Grote, RN
07/21/15 1654	Furosemide (LASIX) intravenous	20 mg slow IV - 2 min.	Karla J Grote, RN
07/21/15 1703	Insulin Aspart (NOVOLOG FLEXPEN) injection	7 units **dual signoff** Karla J Grote/Julia M Box	**Dr. Marczewski, one order 7 units, glucose 477**
07/21/15 1759	Diltiazem (CARDIZEM) tablet 4 times daily	30 mg per G Tube	Karla J Grote, RN
07/21/15 1759	Glucerna 1.0 CAL LIQD every 4 hours	320 mL PEG Tube	Karla J Grote, RN
07/21/15 1907	Albuterol (PROVENTIL) nebulizer	2.5 mg	Phillip R Glenn, RRT
07/21/15 1907	**Budesonide (PULMICORT) nebulizer 2 daily**	**Corticosteroid** .5 mg	Phillip R Glenn, RRT
07/21/15 2114	Ciprofloxacin in D5W IV 2 times per day	200 mL/hr / 60 min	Amanda L Hedberg, RN

07/21/15 2120	Insulin Aspart (NOVOLOG FLEXPEN) injection	5 units **dual signoff**	Tonya Lankford, ARNP Amanda L Hedberg, Amanda J Nees
07/21/15 2120	Insulin detemir (LEVEMIR FLEXPEN) subcutaneous	55 units, **dual signoff**	Sara M Bell, Emily J Lange
07/21/15 2155	Diltiazem (CARDIZEM) tablet 4 times daily	30 mg per G Tube	Amada L Hedberg, RN
07/21/15 2155	Glucerna 1.0 CAL LIQD every 4 hours	320 mL PEG Tube	Amanda L Hedberg, RN
07/21/15 2215	CefTRIAXone (ROCEPHIN) IVPB every 12 hours	100 mL/hr / 30 min.	Amanda L Hedberg, RN

Wednesday July 22, 2015

07/22/15 0212	Glucerna 1.0 CAL LIQD every 4 hours	320 mL PEG Tube	Amanda L Hedberg, RN
07/22/15 0600	Glucerna 1.0 CAL LIQD every 4 hours	320 mL PEG Tube	Jamie L Bloyer RN
07/22/15 0607	Insulin Aspart (NOVOLOG FLEXPEN) injection	4 units **dual signoff**	Tonya Lankford, ARNP, Amanda L Hedberg, Amanda J Nees
07/22/15 0607	Insulin Aspart (NOVOLOG FLEXPEN) injection	4 units dual signoff	Tonya Lankford, ARNP
07/22/15 0754	Albuterol (PROVENTIL) nebulizer	2.5 mg	Phillip R Glenn, RRT
07/22/15 0755	**Budesonide (PULMICORT) nebulizer 2 daily**	**Corticosteroid** .5 mg	Phillip R Glenn, RRT
07/22/15 0915	Furosemide (LASIX) intravenous	20 mg slow IV - 2 min.	Jamie L Bloyer RN

Date/Time	Medication	Dose	Administered by
07/22/15 0915	**MethylPREDISolone sodium succinate injection**	Corticosteroid **40 mg IV 3-5 min**	Jamie L Bloyer RN
07/22/15 0915	Pantoprazole (PROTONIX) injection	40 mg intravenous	Jamie L Bloyer RN
07/22/15 0922	Ciprofloxacin in D5W IV 2 times per day	200 mL/hr / 60 min	Jamie L Bloyer RN
07/22/15 0922	Diltiazem (CARDIZEM) tablet 4 times daily	30 mg per G Tube	Jamie L Bloyer RN
07/22/15 0922	Montelukast (SINGULAIR tablet daily	10 mg per G Tube	Jamie L Bloyer RN
07/22/15 0938	Glucerna 1.0 CAL LIQD every 4 hours	320 mL PEG Tube	Jamie L Bloyer RN
07/22/15 1025	CefTRIAXone (ROCEPHIN) IVPB every 12 hours	100 mL/hr / 30 min.	Jamie L Bloyer RN
07/22/15 1146	Diltiazem (CARDIZEM) tablet 4 times daily	30 mg per G Tube	Jamie L Bloyer RN
07/22/15 1146	Insulin Aspart (NOVOLOG FLEXPEN) injection	5 units **dual signoff**	Tonya Lankford, ARNP Jamie L Bloyer, Julia M Box
07/22/15 1356	Glucerna 1.0 CAL LIQD every 4 hours	320 mL PEG Tube	Jamie L Bloyer RN
07/22/15 1531	Furosemide (LASIX) intravenous	20 mg slow IV - 2 min.	Jamie L Bloyer RN
07/22/15 1802	Albuterol (PROVENTIL) nebulizer	2.5 mg	Phillip R Glenn, RRT
07/22/15 1802	**Budesonide (PULMICORT) nebulizer 2 daily**	**Corticosteroid** 5 mg	Phillip R Glenn, RRT
07/22/15 1803	Diltiazem (CARDIZEM) tablet 4 times daily	30 mg per G Tube	Jamie L Bloyer RN
07/22/15 1803	Glucerna 1.0 CAL LIQD every 4 hours	320 mL PEG Tube	Jamie L Bloyer RN

07/22/15 1803	Insulin Aspart (NOVOLOG FLEXPEN) injection	5 units **dual signoff**	Tonya Lankford, ARNP Jamie L Bloyer, Julia M Box
07/22/15 2119	Ciprofloxacin in D5W IV 2 times per day	200 mL/hr / 60 min	Alison E. Neumann RN
07/22/15 2119	Diltiazem (CARDIZEM) tablet 4 times daily	30 mg per G Tube	Alison E. Neumann RN
07/22/15 2124	Insulin Aspart (NOVOLOG FLEXPEN) injection	1-5 units 4 times daily, **NOT GIVEN**	**Tonya Lankford, ARNP one order 8 units**
07/22/15 2138	Insulin Aspart (NOVOLOG FLEXPEN) injection	8 units **dual signoff**, Tonya Lankford, ARNP	Alison E Neumann, Reena L Hansen
07/22/15 2138	Insulin detemir (LEVEMIR FLEXPEN) subcutaneous	5 units, **dual signoff**	Alison E Neumann, Reena L Hansen
07/22/15 2252	Glucerna 1.0 CAL LIQD every 4 hours	320 mL PEG Tube	Alison E. Neumann RN
07/22/15 2255	CefTRIAXone (ROCEPHIN) IVPB every 12 hours	100 mL/hr / 30 min.	Jamie L Bloyer RN

Thursday July 23, 2015

07/23/15 0221	Glucerna 1.0 CAL LIQD every 4 hours	320 mL PEG Tube	Alison E. Neumann RN
07/23/15 0558	Glucerna 1.0 CAL LIQD every 4 hours	320 mL PEG Tube	Alison E. Neumann RN
07/23/15 0814	**Budesonide (PULMICORT) nebulizer 2 daily**	**Corticosteroid** .5 mg	Patrick Obrien, RT
07/23/15 0816	Albuterol (PROVENTIL) nebulizer	2.5 mg	Patrick Obrien, RT

Date/Time	Medication	Dose/Route	Staff
07/23/15 0836	Insulin Aspart (NOVOLOG FLEXPEN) injection	5 units **dual signoff**,	Tonya Lankford, ARNP Jamie L Bloyer, Kara G Wellington
07/23/15 0842	**MethylPREDISolone sodium succinate injection**	**Corticosteroid 40 mg IV 3-5 min**	Jamie L Bloyer RN
07/23/15 0844	Furosemide (LASIX) intravenous	20 mg slow IV - 2 min.	Jamie L Bloyer RN
07/23/15 0847	Pantoprazole (PROTONIX) injection	40 mg intravenous	Jamie L Bloyer RN
07/23/15 0849	Ciprofloxacin in D5W IV 2 times per day	200 mL/hr / 60 min	Jamie L Bloyer RN
07/23/15 0851	Diltiazem (CARDIZEM) tablet 4 times daily	30 mg per G Tube	Jamie L Bloyer RN
07/23/15 0851	Montelukast (SINGULAIR tablet daily	10 mg per G Tube	Jamie L Bloyer RN
07/23/15 0933	Insulin detemir (LEVEMIR FLEXPEN)subcutaneous	20 units, **dual signoff**	Jamie L Bloyer, Amy J Scheffler
07/23/15 0954	CefTRIAXone (ROCEPHIN) IVPB every 12 hours	100 mL/hr / 30 min.	Alison E. Neumann RN
07/23/15 0954	Glucerna 1.0 CAL LIQD every 4 hours	320 mL PEG Tube	Jamie L Bloyer RN
07/23/15 0954	Insulin detemir (LEVEMIR FLEXPEN)subcutaneous	10 mg (30/30) nightly	Dr. Leszek Marczewski
07/23/15 1131	Insulin Aspart (NOVOLOG FLEXPEN) injection	5 units **dual signoff**,	Tonya Lankford, ARNP, Jamie L Bloyer, Amy J Scheffler
07/23/15 1132	Diltiazem (CARDIZEM) tablet 4 times daily	30 mg per G Tube	Jamie L Bloyer RN
07/23/15 1359	Glucerna 1.0 CAL LIQD every 4 hours	320 mL PEG Tube	Jamie L Bloyer RN

07/23/15 1359	Insulin detemir (LEVEMIR FLEXPEN)subcutaneous	10 mg (30/30) nightly	Dr. Leszek Marczewski
07/23/15 1531	Furosemide (LASIX) intravenous	20 mg slow IV - 2 min.	Jamie L Bloyer RN
07/23/15 1715	Insulin Aspart (NOVOLOG FLEXPEN) injection	5 units **dual signoff**	Tonya Lankford, ARNP,Jamie L Bloyer, Kay Martin
07/23/15 1716	Diltiazem (CARDIZEM) tablet 4 times daily	30 mg per G Tube	Jamie L Bloyer RN
07/23/15 1716	Glucerna 1.0 CAL LIQD every 4 hours	320 mL PEG Tube	Jamie L Bloyer RN
07/23/15 1823	Albuterol (PROVENTIL) nebulizer	2.5 mg	Patrick Obrien, RT
07/23/15 1825	**Budesonide (PULMICORT) nebulizer 2 daily**	**Corticosteroid** .5 mg	Patrick Obrien, RT
07/23/15 2037	Insulin Aspart (NOVOLOG FLEXPEN) injection	1-5 units 4 times daily **NOT GIVEN, blood sugar 504**	**Tonya Lankford, ARNP one order 10 units**
07/23/15 2039	Ciprofloxacin in D5W IV 2 times per day	200 mL/hr / 60 min	Alison E. Neumann RN
07/23/15 2045	Insulin Aspart (NOVOLOG FLEXPEN) injection	10 Units **dual signoff BS** 504	Alison E Neumann, Amanda J Nees
07/23/15 2046	Insulin detemir (LEVEMIR FLEXPEN)subcutaneous	65 units, **dual signoff**	Alison E Neumann, Amanda J Nees
07/23/15 2145	Diltiazem (CARDIZEM) tablet 4 times daily	30 mg per G Tube	Alison E. Neumann RN
07/23/15 2145	Glucerna 1.0 CAL LIQD every 4 hours	320 mL PEG Tube	Alison E. Neumann RN

07/23/15 2218	CefTRIAXone (ROCEPHIN) IVPB every 12 hours	100 mL/hr / 30 min.	Alison E. Neumann RN

Friday July 24, 2015

07/24/15 0215	Glucerna 1.0 CAL LIQD every 4 hours	320 mL PEG Tube	Amanda J Nees, RN
07/24/15 0524	Glucerna 1.0 CAL LIQD every 4 hours	320 mL PEG Tube	Alison E. Neumann RN
07/24/15 0825	Albuterol (PROVENTIL) nebulizer	2.5 mg	Patrick Obrien, RT
07/24/15 0826	**Budesonide (PULMICORT) nebulizer 2 daily**	.5 mg	Patrick Obrien, RT
07/24/15 0905	Insulin Aspart (NOVOLOG FLEXPEN) injection	4 units **dual signoff**	Tonya Lankford, ARNP Jill S Vonahn, Emily J Lange
07/24/15 0908	Insulin detemir (LEVEMIR FLEXPEN)subcutaneous	20 units, **dual signoff**	Jill S Vonahn, Emily J Lange
07/24/15 0915	Ciprofloxacin in D5W IV 2 times per day	200 mL/hr / 60 min	Jill S Vonahn, RN
07/24/15 0917	Furosemide (LASIX) intravenous	20 mg slow IV - 2 min.	Jill S Vonahn, RN
07/24/15 0918	**MethylPREDISolone sodium succinate injection**	**Corticosteroid** 40 mg IV 3-5 min	Jill S Vonahn, RN
07/24/15 0928	Diltiazem (CARDIZEM) tablet 4 times daily	30 mg per G Tube	Jill S Vonahn, RN
07/24/15 0928	Montelukast (SINGULAIR tablet daily	10 mg per G Tube	Jill S Vonahn, RN
07/24/15 0929	Glucerna 1.0 CAL LIQD every 4 hours	320 mL PEG Tube	Jill S Vonahn, RN
07/24/15 0931	Pantoprazole (PROTONIX) injection	40 mg intravenous	Jill S Vonahn, RN

Date/Time	Medication	Dose/Rate	Signoff
07/24/15 1034	CefTRIAXone (ROCEPHIN) IVPB every 12 hours	100 mL/hr / 30 min.	Jill S Vonahn, RN
07/24/15 1057	Insulin Aspart (NOVOLOG FLEXPEN) injection	4 units **dual signoff**	Tonya Lankford, ARNP Jill S Vonahn, Amy J Scheffler
07/24/15 1355	NaCl infusion 0.9%	IV 100 mL/hr	Kay Martin RN
0724/15 1400	Insulin regular (HUMULIN R NOVOLIN R) injection	5 units **dual signoff**	Kay Martin RN, Jill S Vonahn
0724/15 1402	Insulin regular (HUMULIN R NOVOLIN R) injection	5 units **dual signoff**	Kay Martin RN, Jill S Vonahn

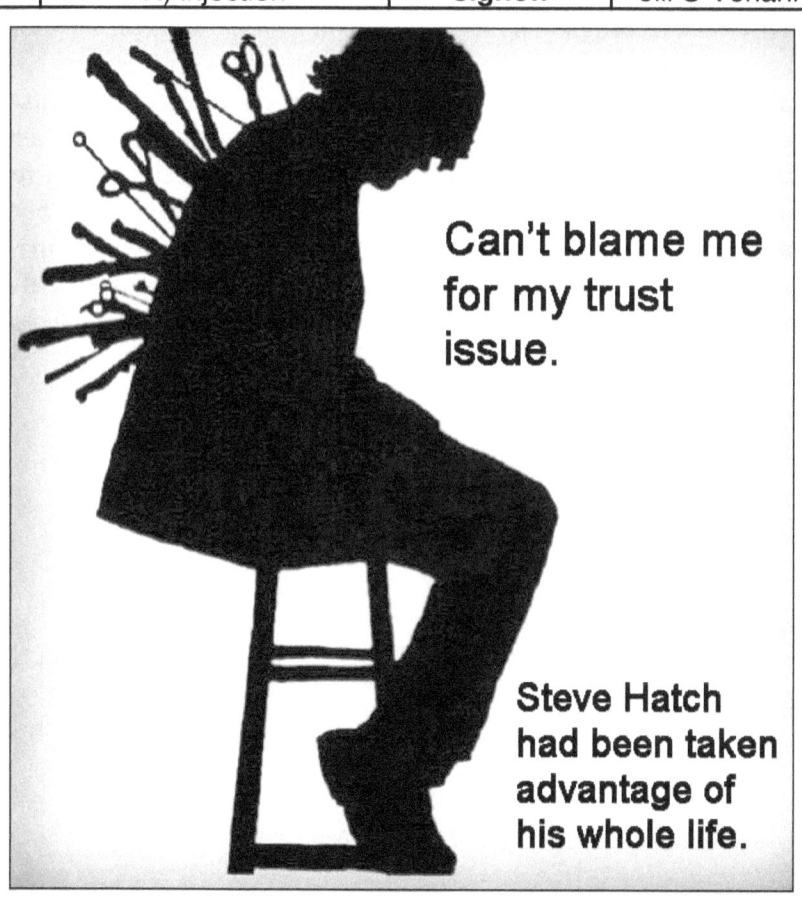

Can't blame me for my trust issue.

Steve Hatch had been taken advantage of his whole life.

Lethal Medications Given During Steve's Final 13 Days

To make the story even more outlandish, Lortab – the same narcotic that has caused Steve's prior aspiration incident, was <u>resumed</u> four days after leaving Loring Hospital and after Steve had been forced into hospice without a terminal illness and without his permission (against Iowa State Laws for admittance into hospice).

Below are the medications by date/times/initials of nurses and include the stomach residue indicating when his stomach had slowed in digesting the liquid nutrients due to the nausea caused by the opioid Lortab. These charts start on 07/28/15 when the Lortab was resumed for pain, four days after he was returned to Blackhawk Life Care into unskilled care/hospice (no stroke therapy).

By 08/03/15 Steve's lungs had filled with vomit and he was gasping for air (air hunger). His digestive system had again shut down causing his stomach unable to digest the liquid feedings filling his stomach resulting in vomiting as noted by the nursing staff who measured the undigested residue from previous feedings. The charts end on 08/06/15 when he took his last breath.

A person who is unable to swallow due to paralyzed neck muscles from a stroke has NO difficulty vomiting stomach contents. The stomach was not paralyzed from the stroke but Steve's swallowing/speech/cough reflux was temporarily not working. All he could do was lay where he had been placed and inhale the liquid as it backed up into this throat. Drowning in your own stomach fluids doesn't happen immediately. It takes hours for the patient gasping for air to finally go unconscious. Drowning is a horrible experience for everyone including a man unable to cry for help.

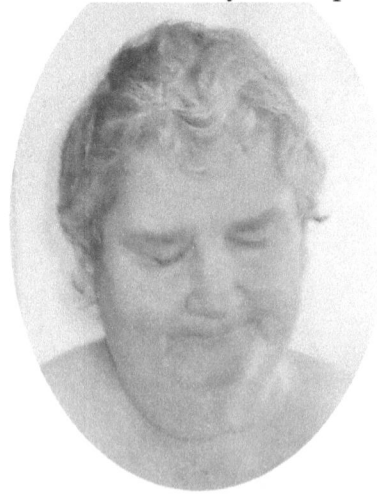

	Narcotics/opioids/morphine administered between 07/28/15 and 08/06/15 that caused Steve's death while in hospice. Included are the stomach residual notations indicating his digestive system had shut down due to the excessive sedation as his lungs slowly filled with fluid. The persons who gave the lethal medications are identified by their initials only, probably hospice employees. The prescriptions came from Loring - Dr. Marczewski (Lortab) and Dr. Pek (Morphine).	
07/28/15 1759	**Lortab Tab 5-325 MG Hydrocodone-Acetaminophen via PEG-tube prn 6 hrs pain**	By JR Effective
07/28/15 2130	Check residual prioir to feeding 6xday	**residual 10**
07/28/15 2200	Pulmicort Suspension 0.5 MG/2ML Budesonide 1 dose inhaled 2xday	By WR
07/29/15 0000	Diltiazem HCl tab 30 mg 1 tab PEG-tube treat hypertension	4 times a day
07/29/15 1330	Check residual prioir to feeding 6xday	**residual 40**
07/29/15 1730	Check residual prioir to feeding 6xday	**residual 40**
07/29/15 1801	**Lortab Tab 5-325 MG Hydrocodone-Acetaminophen via PEG-tube prn 6 hrs pain**	By WR Effective
07/30/15 0130	Check residual prioir to feeding 6xday	**residual 20**
07/30/15 1723	**Lortab Tab 5-325 MG Hydrocodone-Acetaminophen via PEG-tube prn 6 hrs pain**	By WR Effective
07/31/15 0530	Check residual prioir to feeding 6xday	**residual 30**
07/31/15 1730	Check residual prioir to feeding 6xday	**residual 5**
07/31/15 1740	**Lortab Tab 5-325 MG Hydrocodone-Acetaminophen via PEG-tube prn 6 hrs pain**	By WR Effective

08/01/15 0144	**Lortab Tab 5-325 MG Hydrocodone-Acetaminophen via PEG-tube prn 6 hrs pain**	By WR Effective
08/01/15 0530	Check residual prioir to feeding 6xday	**residual 30**
08/01/15 2109	**Lortab Tab 5-325 MG Hydrocodone-Acetaminophen via PEG-tube prn 6 hrs pain**	By WR Effective
08/02/15 0130	Check residual prioir to feeding 6xday	**residual 5**
08/02/15 0352	**Lortab Tab 5-325 MG Hydrocodone-Acetaminophen via PEG-tube prn 6 hrs pain**	By WR Effective
08/02/15 0530	Check residual prioir to feeding 6xday	**residual 10**
08/02/15 0930	Check residual prioir to feeding 6xday	**residual 40**
08/02/15 1330	Check residual prioir to feeding 6xday	**residual 20**
08/02/15 1956	**Lortab Tab 5-325 MG Hydrocodone-Acetaminophen via PEG-tube prn 6 hrs pain**	By WR Effective
08/03/15 0206	**Lortab Tab 5-325 MG Hydrocodone-Acetaminophen via PEG-tube prn 6 hrs pain**	By WR Effective
08/03/15 2009	**Lortab Tab 5-325 MG Hydrocodone-Acetaminophen via PEG-tube prn 6 hrs pain**	by AM **Code 5 see progress notes**
08/03/15 2130	Check residual prioir to feeding 6xday	**residual 10**
08/04/15 0000	Oxyten via NC at 2-5L/NC for sat >90% night	By TB 4L 97
08/04/15 0209	**Lortab Tab 5-325 MG Hydrocodone-Acetaminophen via PEG-tube prn 6 hrs pain**	By AM Effective

08/04/15 1314	**Lortab Tab 5-325 MG Hydrocodone-Acetaminophen via PEG-tube prn 6 hrs pain**	**Code 6 sleeping** By KS Effective
08/04/15 1330	Check residual prioir to feeding 6xday	**residual 20**
08/04/15 1730	Check residual prioir to feeding 6xday	**residual 15**
08/04/15 1900	**Morphine Sulfate Solution 20 MG/ML Give 0.5 ml sublingually (under tongue) every 1 hour as needed for pain/airhunger**	**By WR**
08/04/15 1937	**Lortab Tab 5-325 MG Hydrocodone-Acetaminophen via PEG-tube prn 6 hrs pain**	By WR Effective
08/04/15 2119	**Morphine Sulfate Solution 20 MG/ML Give 0.5 ml sublingually (under tongue) every 1 hour as needed for pain/airhunger**	**by WR**
08/05/15 0530	Check residual prioir to feeding 6xday	**residual 35**
08/05/15 1102	**Morphine Sulfate Solution 20 MG/ML Give 0.5 ml sublingually (under tongue) every 1 hour as needed for pain/airhunger**	by TB **Code 4 Vitals Outside of Parameters for administration**
08/05/15 1330	Check residual prioir to feeding 6xday	**residual 30**
08/05/15 1654	**Morphine Sulfate Solution 20 MG/ML Give 0.5 ml sublingually (under tongue) every 1 hour as needed for pain/airhunger**	**By CK**
08/05/15 1730	Check residual prioir to feeding 6xday	**residual 60**

08/05/15 2122	Atropine -Care Solution (Atropine Sulfate) Give 2 drop by mouth every 4 hours for secretions re **chronic respiratory failure**	CK effective
08/05/15 2122	**Morphine Sulfate Solution 20 MG/ML Give 0.5 ml sublingually (under tongue) every 1 hour as needed for pain/airhunger**	**By CK**
08/05/15 2130	Check residual prioir to feeding 6xday	**residual 30**
08/06/15 0130	Check residual prioir to feeding 6xday	**residual 70**
08/06/15 0230	**Steven Lee Hatch passed away after his heart and lungs again filled with stomach fluid from Lortab which caused vomiting and stomach fluid residue indicating his digestion system had again shut down due to the Lortab.**	

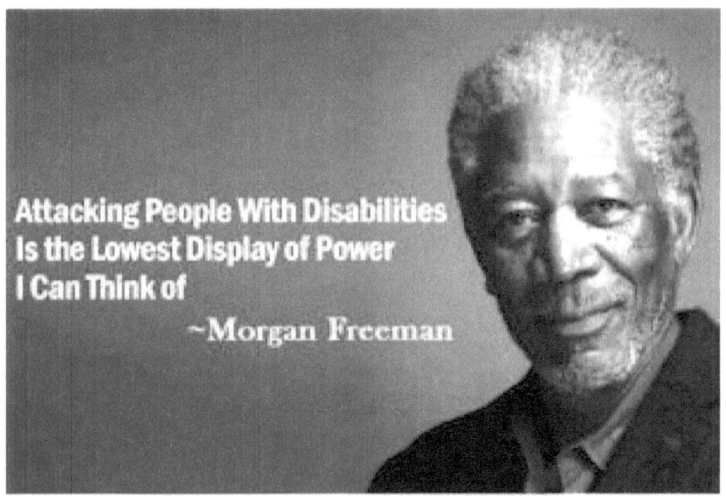

By Marlys J. Waters

Doctors Who Worked Against Steve's Best Interest Leading to His Death.

Dr. Shaheer Ahmed Siddiqui, Mercy Medical Center

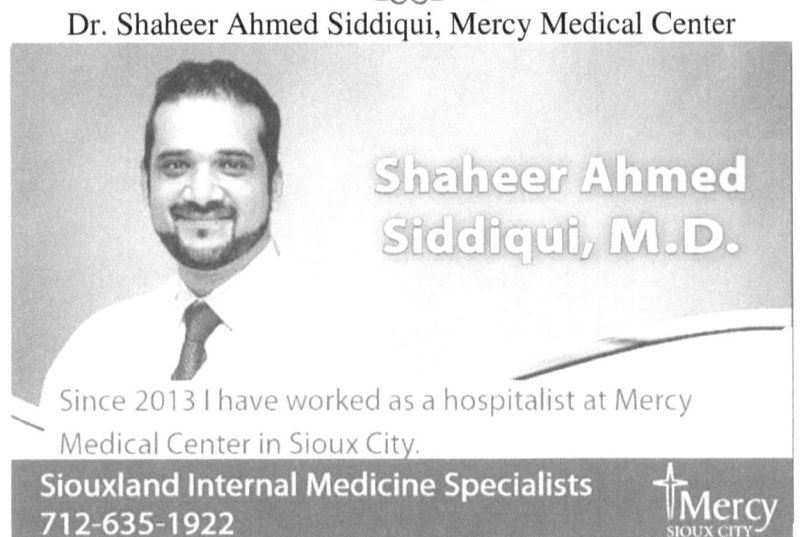

Dr. Shaheer Ahmed Siddiqui, MD., Mercy Medical Center, Sioux City, IA 712 635-1922

06/23/15 Jpg 60 ☹Dr. Siddiqui examined Steve in the stroke ward in the morning as indications of aspiration first started. Steve was receiving oxygen at 4LPM (very high volume) delivered by an OxyMask.

06/23/15 Jpg 61 ☹ Stable, alert, failed swallow evaluation so needs PEG tube (into stomach).

06//27/15 Jpg 95: ☹ Patient is probably having ileus (vomiting). *[Sedatives/opioids cause vomiting, very dangerous for a person that can't swallow. MJW]*

06/24/15 ☹ After Steve had been taken to ICU due to aspiration incident, Dr. Siddiqui consulted with Dr. Elizabeth McInerney and asked the estranged brother to come in to discuss the needed PEG tube for easier feeding and to also give permission for palliative (comfort, hospice) care since there was little chance of Steve's recovery (their opinion after treating him for two days).

Brother Don Hatch refused to sign Steve into hospice for comfort care and out of stroke therapy/rehabilitation but he did sign the DNR order (do not resuscitate) in the event of cardio/pulmonary cessation (if both his heart and lungs stopped).

The Killing Field Known as Hospice

Dr. Elizabeth McInerney, Mercy Medical Center,

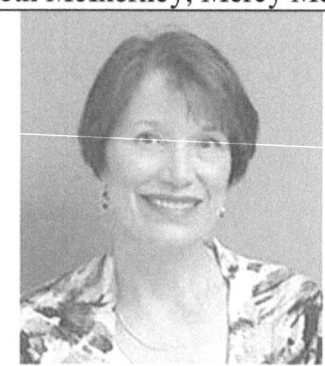

Dr. Elizabeth A McInerney, MD,
Family Medicine Sioux City, IA,
Office Address
Mercy Medical Center
801 5th Street
Sioux City, IA 51101
Phone:(712) 279-2010

Dr. Elizabeth A. McInerney, Family Medicine, Sioux City, IA, Office: Mercy Medical Center, 801 5th St, Sioux City, IA 51101, Phone (712) 279-2010

06/24/15 ☹ Dr. Sidduqui consulted with Dr. Elizabeth McInerney and asked the estranged brother to come in to discuss the needed PEG tube for easier feeding and to also give permission for palliative (comfort, hospice) care since there was little chance of Steve's recovery (their opinion after treating him for two days).

06/26/15 Jpg 43: ☹ He remains deeply encephalopathic (stroke damage) and minimally responsive. *[He fainted from lack of oxygen after his lungs filled up with stomach fluids over 24 hours plus is probably sedated so he doesn't fight the BIPAP air mask.MJW]*

06/26/2015 Jpg 45: ☹ His prognosis is grim for regaining independence; we would continue to encourage family to consider comfort care (palliative/hospice).

07/06/15 Jpg 128 ☹ Dr. Elizabeth A. McInerney "Palliative care is going to sign off the case at this point. Family signed DNR but decided for tube feeding and nursing home option. His prognosis remains extremely guarded. He has had several strokes *[Not True. MJW]*. He is in atrial fib and has severe to critical aortic stenosis. He has no pain or distress.

By Marlys J. Waters

Dr. Thomas R. Murphy, Affiliated with Mercy Medical Center, Sioux City, Iowa

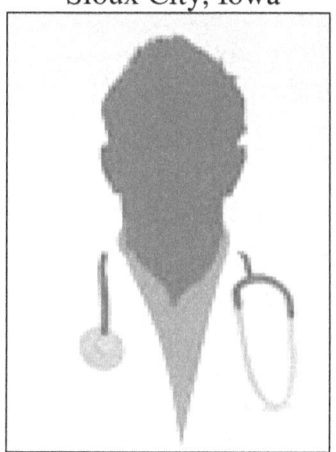

Dr. Thomas R Murphy MD, has 25 years experience. He is currently practicing at 1200 6Th Ave N in St Cloud, MN. as a Doctor of Critical Care (Intensivists).

Dr. Thomas obtained its degree in Critical Care (Intensivists) from New York Medical College in the year 1993. Doctor Murphy has been awarded more than 9 times for top-notch work in Critical Care (Intensivists) field. He is an affiliated MD in Healtheast St John's Hospital and other Hospitals. He accepts patients Centracare Clinic Health organization.

Dr. Thomas Murphy is a pulmonologist in Bozeman. He diagnoses and treats patients who suffer from respiratory or breathing problems such as asthma and COPD

Hospital Affiliation of Dr. Thomas Murphy:

1. Healtheast St John'S Hospital
2. Healtheast St. Joseph's Hospital
3. **Mercy Medical Center-Sioux City**
4. Healtheast Woodwinds Hospital
5. Marian Health Center-smhc
6. St Cloud Hospital
7. Bozeman Deaconess Health Services

06/24/15 Jpg 40 ☹ Patient is morbidly obese, follows with Dr. Stewart. Patient had a respiratory event secondary to aspiration of NG tube feedings and dysphagia *[unable to swallow. MJW]*.

06/24/2015 Jpg 42: ☹He is in acute respiratory failure. Hopefully can wean BIPAP overnight.

06/25/2015 Jpg 82: ☹Recommends a trach, beneficial to make him a do not resuscitate. *[A trach through his throat into his lungs is barbaric. He really needs a PEG tube into the stomach for safer feedings and medications. MJW]*

06/26/15 Jpg 92: ☹We are having some issues with him waking up *[Opioids/Fentanyl slow down respiration on people with COPD. MJW]*

06/27/15 Jpg 103: ☹Looks like tube feedings that he aspirated. Keep head of bed elevated. Brother not ready to make Steve comfort care at this time (hospice). **"I would recommend not bringing him back down to the Intensive Care Unit".***[That statement goes against EMTALA that was enacted in 1986 under Section 1867 of the Social Security Act. It states any individual who comes to the emergency department must be provided an appropriate medical screening examination. That is also proof that just because brother Don Hatch signed a DNR on 06/27/15 order that Mercy Hospital plans to not even attempt to treat him if he aspirates again which was their negligence in the first place. The DNR order is only valid if the heart AND lungs have stopped. MJW]*

Dr. Jon A. Peacock, Mercy Medical Center, Sioux City, Iowa

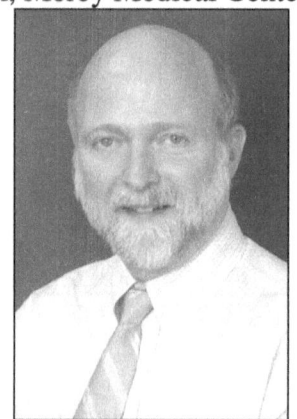

Dr. Jon A. Peacock 06/25/15 Jpg 75: ☹Started FentaNYL for pain (a dangerous opioid/narcotic) and Haldol (Antipsychotic to decrease excitement in the brain.) *[Very dangerous for persons with breathing problems. MJW]*

06/27/15 Jpg 102: ☹Intubated in ICU. Had slow heart rates yesterday. Now is "Do Not Resuscitate" status. Is going to be treated by the palliative care team. *[NO, he is NOT going to be put into hospice and treated by the palliative care team just 4 days after the stroke. MJW]* No change in stroke abnormalities.

Dr. Robert Stewart, Affiliated with Mercy Medical Center, Sioux City, Iowa

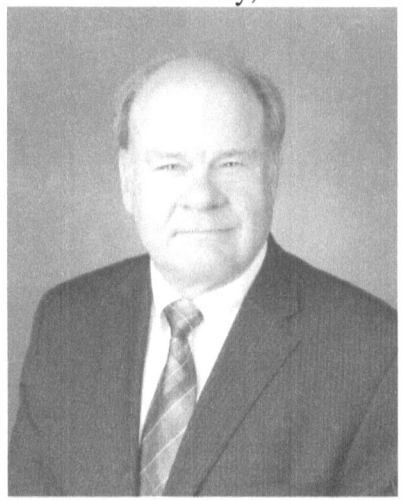

Dr. Robert Stewart. 2730 Pierce St, Suite 401, Sioux City, IA 51104, (712) 255-8827

Specializes in Critical Care Medicine, Board certified in Critical Care Medicine, Internal Medicine, Pulmonary Disease and Sleep Medicine. Specialties: Critical Care Medicine, Pulmonology, Sleep Medicine.

Dr. Robert Stewart is an internist affiliated with multiple hospitals in the area, including Mercy Hospital and Mercy Medical Center-Sioux City. He received his medical degree from University of Iowa Carver College of Medicine and has been in practice for more than 20 years. He is one of 15 at Mercy Medical Center-Sioux City who specializes in Internal Medicine.

[☹ This is the doctor that prescribed Zafirlukast (ACCOLATE) for Steve's asthma in 2013 and which caused 2 years of unexplained gastro/intestinal bleeding requiring multiple hospital stays, multiple endoscopy/coloscopy exams, and many blood transfusions. MJW]

The Killing Field Known as Hospice
Dr. Marczewski, Loring Hospital, and Blackhawk plotting to get Steve Hatch into Hospice 7/07/15 -08/06/15

Dr. Leszak Marczewski, Loring Hospital, Sac City, Iowa

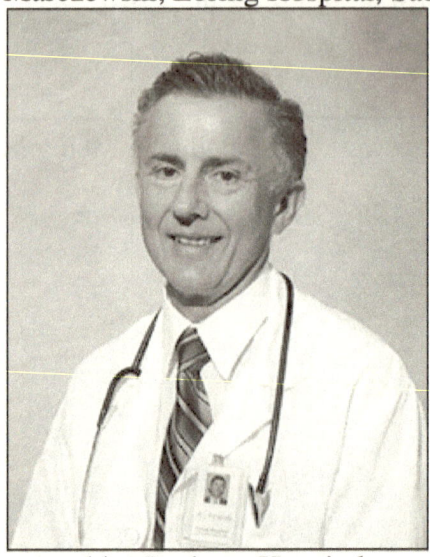

Dr. Leszak Marczewski, Loring Hospital, prescribed Lortab on 7/10/2015 for use by nurses at Blackhawk as needed every 6 hours for pain.

---

801 Prescription Drugs ISBN 0-915099-086-1 — PAIN AND ARTHRITIS / 367

Acetaminophen with Hydrocodone Bitartrate
Brand names: *Anexsia, Bancap HC, Hydrocet, Lorcet, Lorcet Plus, Lortab, Panacet, Vicodin, Vicodin ES* **(Generic available)**

What this drug does for you:
This drug combines acetaminophen with a narcotic painkiller very similar to codeine. Narcotics relieve pain by depressing your central nervous system.

Possible side effects of this drug:
- This drug most often causes dizziness, drowsiness, and nausea. It can also cause constipation, mood changes, mental clouding, and difficulty urinating. One of the most dangerous side effects of hydrocodone at high doses is slow or irregular breathing.

Special warnings:
- Hydrocodone suppresses the cough reflex, so people with lung disease should take this drug with caution.
- This drug should be used with caution by people with head injuries, as it may increase fluid pressure on the brain.
- Older people and people with liver or kidney damage, an underactive thyroid, Addison's disease, or an enlarged prostate should take this drug with caution.

Possible food and drug interactions:
- If you take this drug along with alcohol or a drug that depresses your nervous system, such as tranquilizers, antihistamines, or muscle relaxants, the combination may dangerously depress your nervous system.

. This occurred three days after Steve's arrival at Blackhawk where he had been admitted into their Skilled Care for stroke rehabilitation/therapy paid by Medicare for up to 90 days. This dangerous narcotic is absolutely NOT to be used for an elderly stroke resident and would eventually lead to his death. There can be only one reason it was prescribed, -- a collusion between nurses/administrators at Blackhawk and Dr. Marczewski to work toward getting Steve Hatch OUT of skilled nursing care (stroke rehab) and into hospice.

On 07/10/15 Steve Hatch was alert. Stroke therapy had started. He had no pain or other critical care needs on that day. This medication caused over four days of vomiting from stomach irritation which he inhaled into his lungs since he was unable to swallow/cough. This was direct torture of a disabled man who couldn't fight back. I can not fathom people who are so despicable to purposely cause a paralyzed man to aspirate his own vomit while being ignored for 4 days over 24 hour Mitt checks indicating vomit.

From Wikipedida: "**Waterboarding** is a form of water torture in which water is poured over a cloth covering the face and breathing passages of an immobilized captive, causing the individual to experience the sensation of drowning. Ordinarily, the water is poured intermittently so as to prevent death during torture; however, if the water is poured uninterruptedly it will lead to death by asphyxia. Besides death, waterboarding can cause extreme pain, damage to lungs, and brain damage from oxygen deprivation."

Allowing a disabled man to lay flat on his back in bed over four days as his lungs slowly fill up with stomach fluid (vomit) while he is heavily sedated is the lowest form of torture imaginable.

Steve Hatch was left laying in bed at Blackhawk Life Care for over 4 days starting on 07/13/15 as his lungs were again slowly filling up with his own vomit, a side effect of Lortab in combination with other medications. The Blackhawk Life Care medical records show an hourly mitt check where Steve was using the white protective cover over his left hand to try to clear his mouth of vomit, some days up to 8 continuous hours, an obvious unmonitored side effect of one (or more) medications that were ignored.

After Steve was having noticeable trouble breathing, he was taken to Loring Hospital by ambulance for treatment of aspiration pneumonia on the evening of 07/16/15. The strong narcotic Lortab/Norco which Dr. Marczewski had prescribed for use at Blackhawk Life Care Center to be used at their discretion every 6 hours for pain was suddenly stopped during his stay at Loring Hospital. Guess all his pain suddenly disappeared??? Or maybe there was NO pain in the first place???

I do not know who at Blackhawk Life Care Center asked Dr. Marczewski to prescribe a strong opioid for pain. Maybe it was Dr. Marczewski's idea? His name seems to come up a lot when there is a change of condition or care of Steve. You will see from the medication records that what happens next is just as ludricrous. Steve didn't have a chance to fight back once he was forced into hospice.

After Steve had been released from Loring Hospital on 07/24/15 (in hospice) for successful treatment of aspiration pneumonia caused by Lortab, Dr. Marczewski authorized Hospice nurses at Blackhawk Life Care Center to resume Lortab on 07/28/15 which caused the third and final aspiration incident.

☹ 5-325 MG (Hydrocodone - Acetaminophen) 1 tablet via PEG-Tube every 6 hours as needed for pain. It is a strong narcotic that can slow or stop the patient's breathing. It is not recommended for use by people with a history of head injury, brain tumor, stroke; Asthma, COPD, heart disorders or other breathing disorders. (Steve had all these disorders.)

Dr. Leszak Marczewski knew what he was doing, Steve was now in Hospice, no one would know why he died just four days before the Guardianship court date where he would have been taken home to not only recover from the stroke but to prove Steve had no terminal illness.

When Steve had been taken to Loring Hospital on 07/16/15 – 07/24/15 for aspiration pneumonia, Dr. Leszak Marczewski was the attending physician who had originally prescribed Lortab on 07/10/15 to be used prn at Blackhawk Life Care center for pain before Steve was put into hospice..

However at Loring hospital on 07/16/15 the Lortab was immediately stopped, probably because Dr. Marczewski knew it had caused the aspiration pneumonia and that Loring might have questioned its use on their premises and in their medical records which were available to all medical staff at Loring Hospital. Dr. Marczewski's Lortab prescription could not be easily obtained from Blackhawk Life Care records as the managing company

The doctor's names in this book broke state laws by forcing Steve into hospice without his knowledge or permission. Dr. Marczewski tried to imply that Steve was comatose, in a vegative state as if that was going to make his decision any more legal. The nurses and therapists stated on most of their records that Steve was able to respond with yes/no to their questions including the day when he was placed into hospice and on subsequent days.

Dr. Hugh F. Leigh, Loring Hospital, Sac City, Iowa

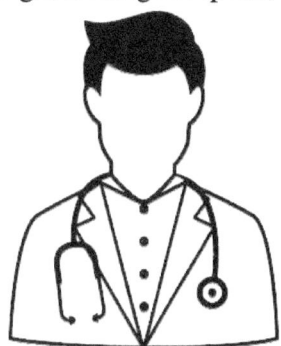

Hugh F Leigh, MD is a Medicare enrolled "Family Medicine" physician in Neligh, Nebraska. He graduated from medical school in 1973 and has 43 years of diverse experience with area of expertise as General Practice. He is a member of the group practice Neligh Clinic Llc and his current practice location is 902 Goldenrod Ln, Neligh, Nebraska NE 68756-2000. You can reach his office (for appointments etc.) via phone at (402) 887-4803.

Hugh F Leigh is licensed to practice in Iowa (license number 23239). He accepts Medicare assignments (which means he accepts the Medicare-approved amount; you will not be billed for any more than the Medicare deductible and coinsurance) and his NPI Number is 1417047176.

He accepts temporary appointments at these affililated hospitals:
- Floyd Valley Hospital, Le mars, IA. Critical Access Hospital
- **Loring Hospital, Sac city, IA. Critical Access Hospital**
- Dallas County Hospital, Perry, IA. Critical Access Hospital

Dr. Hugh Leigh was the Attending Physician at Loring Hospital on the afternoon of 07/24/15 after Dr. Marczewski had disappeared. ☹ He signed the "Certification of Terminal Illness" form to place Steve into Hospice.

He examined and treated Steve Hatch when he was returned to Loring Hospital ER on 7/24/2015 at 3:51 after it had been determined that Steve was unresponsive upon arrival at Blackhawk Life Care Center after the van ride. Steve was <u>conscious</u> when the Certification Form was signed.

Dr. Hugh Leigh did not know about the van ride. It is illegal to place a conscious person into hospice without their permission and without a terminal illness. Fainting from lack of oxygen is not a terminal illness. A recent stroke is not a terminal illness.

Dr. Michael Slattery, McFarland Clinic, Carroll, Iowa
Representing Gentiva Hospice on 07/24/15

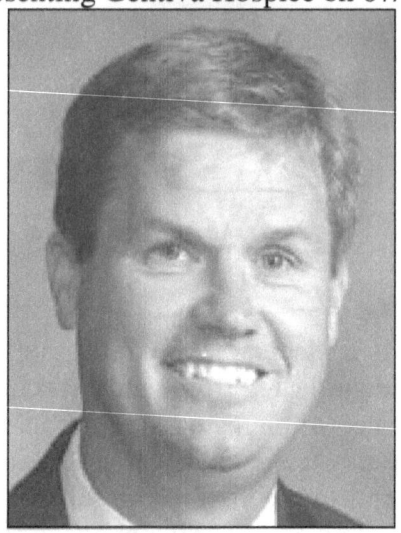

☹ Dr. Michael Slattery, the physician representing hospice, signed (verbally by phone via Vera Reyes RN) on the Gentiva Hospice Physician Certification of Terminal Illness on 7/24/2015. He did not examine Steve Hatch. It is illegal to place a conscious person into hospice without their permission and without a terminal illness.

☹Vera Reyes RN, signed verbal certification of Dr. Michael Slattery's name on the Hospice Physician Certification of Terminal Illness. She also noted "Patient in bed during assessment, awakens to his name, speech mumbled except able to relay yes/no to questions. Lethargic, dozes off very easily."

Dr. Zolten Pek, Loring Hospital, Sac City, Iowa

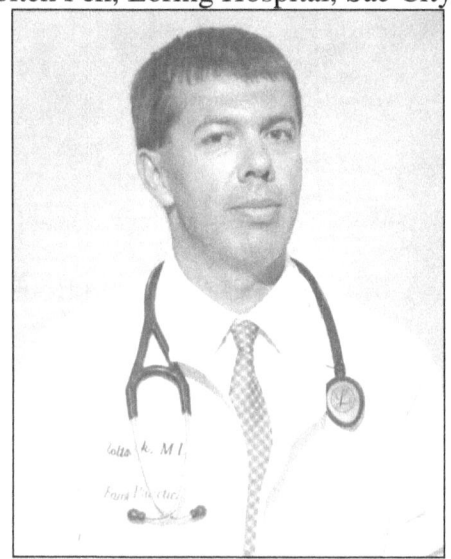

☹ Dr. Zolten Pek had been Steve Hatch's primary physician. His name is listed as Attending Physician on the Gentiva Hospice "Initial Certification of Terminal Illness" dated 07/24/15, the day Steve was forced into hospice after passing out during a van ride without oxygen on a hot summer day.

☹ On 08/04/15 Dr. Pek wrote a prescription for Morphine prn (as needed hourly) based on recommendations from Hospice Staff complaining that Steve was suffering from air-hunger (gasping for air like a fish out of water) without an examination of Steve. The seven days of opioids (Lortab prescribed by Dr. Marczewski on 07/28/15) were causing Steve's lungs to fill with fluid again just like they did between 07/10/15 – 07/16/15 causing the air-hunger reflex (gasping for air).

☹ 08/04/15 - 08/05/2015 Morphine Sulfate (Concentrate) Solution 20 MG/ML. Give .5 ml sublingually every 1 hour as needed for pain/airhunger. *[Morphine caused Steve Hatch to quit breathing and his heart to stop on 08/06/15 at 0230 in the early morning. MJW]*

What is an ARNP? :An advanced registered nurse practitioner (ARNP) is a registered nurse who completes a graduate-level educational program. An ARNP can have primary responsibility for patient care. ARNPs practice independently and also may work with physicians and other health care professionals.

The licensed ARNP may:
- Examine patients and establish diagnoses by patient history, physical examination and other assessments
- Admit, manage and discharge patients to and from health care facilities
- Order, collect, perform and interpret diagnostic tests
- Manage health care by identifying, developing, implementing and evaluating a plan of care and treatment for patients
- Prescribe therapies and medical equipment
- Prescribe medications when necessary
- Refer patients to other health care providers, services or facilities

---

Tonya J. Lankford, ARNP, Loring Hospital, Sac City, Iowa

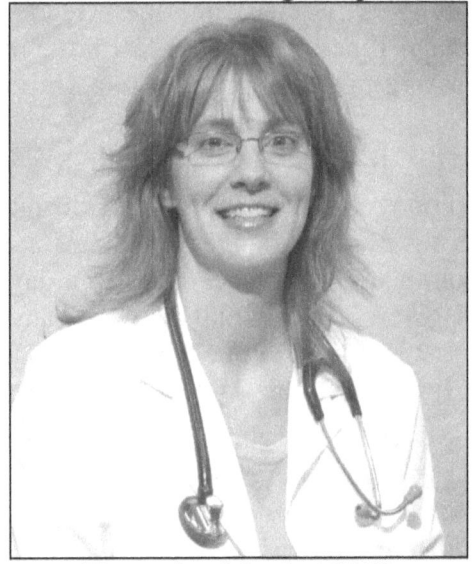

Tonya Lankford, ARNP

Tonya Lankford appeared to have been called in to assist with administering insulin between 07/21/15 - 07/24/15 during the 4-day fiasco when Steve Hatch was being given an extraordinarily high quantity of unnecessary medications during the 2nd 4-days that he had been at Loring Hospital. Maybe she can give some insight on why Steve was given so much medication over 4 days.

Steve had been successfully treated for aspiration pneumonia at Loring between 07/16/15 – 07/20/15 and was discharged (on the medical records) to be taken back to Blackhawk Life Care into skilled Care for stroke rehabilitation. But he never left the hospital.

Instead he was readmitted (still in good shape – alert with clear lungs per stethoscope) and was kept an additional 4 days where a large quantity of medications were suddenly ordered and administered to him causing him to decline in awareness and wrecked havoc with his diabetes (high steroids for breathing work against treatment for diabetes.

The full medical records (not included in this book) will show the difference between curative medications (good) administered 07/16/15-07/20/15 and those given 07/21/15-07/24/15 (bad) concluding with Dr. Marczewski indicating on 07/24/15 that Steve was "comatose" and discharged him from Loring for a van ride back to Blackhawk Life Care Center for stroke rehabilitation. You know what happened after the van ride on 07/24/15.

The "duel signoff" by Tonya Lankford and others appears to be required when unusually high doses of medications are being given requiring more than one nurse to approve the dosage. Tonya Lankford's name was included on those listed below as "<u>triple</u> signoff". That is pretty serious when two nurses ask for a third person (an ARNP) to validate medication orders from a doctor (attending physician Dr. Marczewski??).

I believe that Tonya Lankford can easily indicate who was in charge of giving the medication orders. She can also indicate which nurses called her in to give backup to the medication orders to protect themselves for the dangerously high blood sugar count which required such high and frequent doses of insulin. My guess is the attending physician Dr. Leszak Marczewski purposely attempted to get Steve unconscious so he could be put into hospice "no questions asked" and so Blackhawk Life Care would accept Steve into their unskilled care program.

The use of steroids (Corticosteroids) can cause significantly high blood sugar levels. These hormones decrease the effectiveness of insulin and make your liver dump more glucose into your bloodstream. Some people can have blood sugars as high as 400 mg/dL to 500 mg/dL while taking steroids"

Next are the dates/times when Tonya Lankford was the third person present to approve the extra doses of insulin needed to attempt to control the sky-rocking blood sugar count (indicated with triple signoff).

- 07/21/15 2120 triple signoff 5 units insulin.
- 07/22/15 0607 triple signoff 4 units insulin
- 07/22/15 0607 single signoff 4 units insulin
- 07/22/15 1146 triple signoff 5 units insulin
- 07/22/15 1803 triple signoff 5 units insulin
- 07/22/15 2124 ~~NOT GIVEN~~ 8 units insulin
- 07/22/15 2138 triple signoff 8 units insulin
- 07/23/15 0836 triple signoff 5 units insulin
- 07/23/15 1131 triple signoff 5 units insulin
- 07/23/15 1715 triple signoff 5 units insulin
- 07/23/15 2037 ~~NOT GIVEN~~ 10 units insulin
- 07/24/15 0905 triple signoff 4 units insulin
- 07/24/15 1057 triple signoff 4 units insulin
- 07/24/15 1400 dual signoff 5 units insulin
- 07/24/15 1402 dual signoff 5 units insulin

Use of corticosteroids to treat COPD (asthma/breathing problems) can lead to higher than normal blood glucose levels. This is what happened to Steve Hatch to cause his mental and physical condition to decline between 07/20/15 – 07/24/15 so that the semi-conscious man could be forced into hospice and no one would question that he was obviously dying (of something).

It worked. Steve was forced into hospice on 07/24/15 and was dead 13 days later from opioids and Morphine. Tonya Lankford may be able to give some insight of what she witnessed and who participated in the over-medication between 07/20/15 – 07/24/15.

By Marlys J. Waters
The Admittance into Gentiva Hospice 07/24/15 Was a Profitable move for them
Gentiva (Kindred) Hospice, 712 792-2191
831 N Griffith RD
Carroll, IA 51401

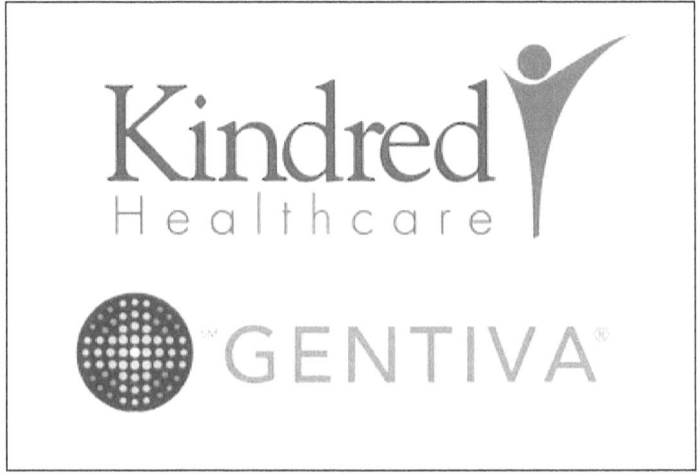

On 07/24/15 Steve Hatch was put into hospice after fainting due to hypoxia (lack of oxygen to the brain) following a van ride. Dr. Marczewski had earlier told brother Don Hatch that Steve was failing indicating he was dying and should be put into hospice. Don said he would think about it.

Steve Hatch had been successfully treated for aspiration pneumonia and was ready to be released from Loring on 06/20/15 but Blackhawk didn't want him back for skilled nursing care, they would only accept him if he was in hospice. So Steve Hatch was kept at Loring for an additional four days and given intense corticosteroids treatments for breathing using nebulizers and oral medications between 07/20/15 – 07/24/15.

Steroids work against diabetes meds which caused Steve's blood sugar to skyrocket and was uncontrollable with normal insulin and required multiple nusrses to work in pairs to signoff the excessive quantity of insulin. (See previous chapter). This excess medication caused Steve's physical and mental psyche to detioriate. Steve was released from Loring after Dr. Marczewski noted on the medical records that he was comatose and placed in a van, sitting upright, without external oxygen for the 30 minute ride to Blackhawk Life Care Center.

As expected by Dr. Marczewski, Steve arrived at Blackhawk unconscious and was taken back to Loring Hospital so that the brother could be convinced that Steve was really dying. It worked, Dr. Leigh was now working in the ER, say (or had been told) that "family was considering hospice". The brother came in and signed Steve into hospice. Heidi Pickhinke Schultus from hospice signed the form. Dr. Michael Slatttery representing the hospice physician also signed the form along with Dr. Leigh who had never seen Steve before.

Steve had regained consciousness during the ambulance ride back to the hospital but no one asked him if he wanted to be placed into hospice even through he had told Heidi Pickhinke Schultus on 074/08/15 that he did NOT want to be put into hospice. I guess she didn't want to ask him this time because he might refuse again.

So nothing further needed to be done after tests were run on Steve's lungs, blood oxygen, and Steve was still conscious, Dr. Leigh signed the hospice document and Steve was returned to Blackhawk by ambulance with oxygen and put into unskilled care with no stroke therapy required.

Hospice was happy because they would be paid for full-time nursing of the dying man, Blackhawk was happy to be paid for furnishing him, baths, bedding changes, and not much else. Dr. Marczewski was VERY HAPPY to never have to treat Steve Hatch again since he would not be allowed back into Loring Hospital since there was a DNR (Do Not Resuscitate) order still active from Mercy Medical Center.

Hospice used Dr. Marczewski's prescription on 07/28/15 for Lortab to restart the process to get Steve's lung filled back up with vomit. They just needed to get him dead before Marlys Water's court date of 08/10/15 when she would take him home and discover he wasn't really dying of anything.

A prescription from Dr. Pek on 08/04/15 for Morphine every 1 hours as needed for pain stopped his heart and lungs on 08/06/15 right on schedule.

By Marlys J. Waters
About the Author

Marlys J. Waters was born and raised on a farm southeast of Nemaha, Iowa. After graduating from Crestland Community School (Early and Nemaha) in 1963, she attended Iowa State University and Drake University, and stayed thirty years in the Ames and Des Moines area

Marlys returned to her hometown of Nemaha, Iowa in 1993 to care for her parents. She now runs a used music and book store, and hosts local websites. She runs "Power of the Pen Publishing" out of Nemaha, Iowa. She also writes books and compiles music books for resale.

Marlys Waters and Steve Hatch grew up on farms four miles apart. While he was three years younger and they knew each other as teenagers, they didn't socialize other than riding horses on the same gravel roads with the same neighbor kids.

Their grandmothers belonged to the same neighborhood Grandmother's Club. It was natural for Marlys and Steve to connect after retirement age when they were again living within miles of each other and shared the same background, knew the same local history, and both loved anything to do with farming and livestock.

Also they were both single without children and had a bright future together as a couple.

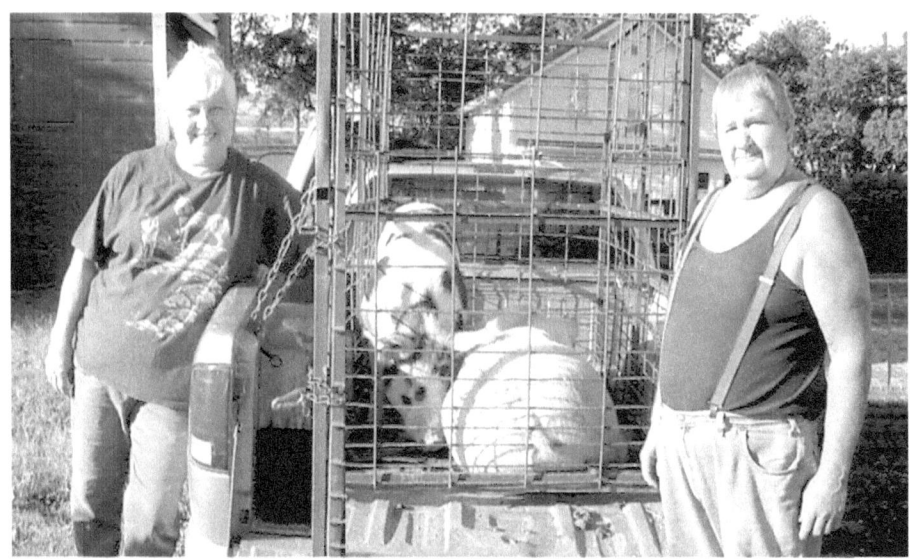

www.ingramcontent.com/pod-product-compliance
Lightning Source LLC
Chambersburg PA
CBHW020456220526
45464CB00002B/1011